ON THE CAUSES OF FEVERS (1839)

The Henry E. Sigerist Supplements to the
Bulletin of the History of Medicine

New Series, no. 9
Editor: Caroline Hannaway

Henry E. Sigerist, recruited by William H. Welch to be director of the Johns Hopkins Institute of the History of Medicine, was the founder of the *Bulletin of the History of Medicine* and also of the first series of supplements, which extended from 1943 to 1951. It was Sigerist's resolve that the *Bulletin* should provide the organ not only of the Johns Hopkins Institute but also of the American Association for the History of Medicine, and to this day it subserves both functions. It is therefore eminently suitable that the new series should bear the founder's name and perpetuate his scholarly interests. These interests were so broad and so varied that the supplements will recognize no narrow limits in range of theme and will publish historical essays of greater scope than the *Bulletin* itself can accommodate. It is not too much to hope that in time the Sigerist supplements will help to extend the purview of medical history.

Other Books in the New Series

1. *Almost Persuaded: American Physicians and Compulsory Health Insurance, 1912–1920,* by Ronald L. Numbers
2. *William Harvey and His Age: The Professional and Social Context of the Discovery of the Circulation,* edited by Jerome J. Bylebyl
3. *The Clinical Training of Doctors: An Essay of 1793* by Philippe Pinel, edited and translated by Dora B. Weiner
4. *Times, Places, and Persons: Aspects of the History of Epidemiology,* edited by Abraham Lilienfeld
5. *When the Twain Meet: The Rise of Western Medicine in Japan,* by John Z. Bowers
6. *A Celebration of Medical History: The Fiftieth Anniversary of the Johns Hopkins Institute of the History of Medicine and the Welch Medical Library,* edited by Lloyd G. Stevenson
7. *Teaching the History of Medicine at a Medical Center,* edited by Jerome J. Bylebyl
8. *Letters of Edward Jenner, and Other Documents Concerning the Early History of Vaccination,* edited by Genevieve Miller

ON THE CAUSES
OF FEVERS (1839)

by

William Budd

Edited by

DALE C. SMITH

THE JOHNS HOPKINS UNIVERSITY PRESS

Baltimore and London

The Johns Hopkins University Press, Baltimore, Maryland 21218
The Johns Hopkins Press Ltd., London

Library of Congress Cataloging in Publication Data

Budd, William, 1811-1880.
On the causes of fevers (1839).

(The Henry E. Sigerist supplements to the Bulletin of
the history of medicine; new ser., no. 9)
Includes bibliographical references and index.
1. Typhoid fever — Great Britain. 2. Typhoid fever —
Ireland. I. Smith, Dale C. II. Title. III. Series.
[DNLM: 1. Typhoid — Etiology. 2. Typhoid — Occurrence —
England. WC 270 B927o]
RC194.G7B84   1984   616.9'272   83-23875
ISBN 0-8018-3166-0

CONTENTS

PREFACE

In December 1839 William Budd submitted an unsuccessful essay in competition for the 1840 Thackeray Prize of the Provincial Medical and Surgical Association (forerunner of the British Medical Association). The subject chosen by the association was the study of the causes and spread of common continued fevers in Great Britain. William Budd's essay was not an influential historical document; it was in fact read by relatively few people. It is important because its author continued to investigate the subject of typhoid fever and was, in large measure, responsible for the increased concern over the contagious nature of disease in Victorian Britain. The 1839 essay is the first, admittedly immature, expression of his views — views that grew under the stimulus of further research until published in a more complete form in 1859. It is clear that the 1839 essay was a working document used in the preparation of Budd's published work.

An introduction and afterword are included to assist the reader in understanding Budd's thoughts in 1839 and the state of fever studies in the early nineteenth century. The editorial commentary in the essay itself is, therefore, generally confined to the provision of complete references to essay material. The footnotes, numbered sequentially in each chapter, are the creation of the editor. These footnotes are primarily composed of three sets of notes to the manuscript essay. The first, a numerical series in parentheses, consists of Budd's original footnotes to the 1839 essay, which are numbered in two sequences, (1)–(42) in chapters 1 and 2, and (1)–(4) in chapter 3. Two of Budd's original footnotes were marked by asterisks; these are noted here by (*), and they occur in chapter 2 between notes (10) and (11) and notes (17) and (18). The second set of footnotes is made up of those marked with symbols — daggers, †, and asterisks, * — which represent later additions to the text, generally written on the back of the previous page. Daggers, †, mark material presumably added by Budd himself; asterisks, *, material added by others. At least three hands are represented: those of John

Conolly, John Forbes, and Thomas Jeffreys, the judges appointed by the Provincial Medical and Surgical Association to judge the essays submitted for the Thackeray Prize. Their notes are usually signed with initials, but some notes are unsigned. Some of the unsigned notes are clearly by John Forbes; others may represent a fourth hand. Most such notes were added between 1840 and 1843, but some were added as late as the 1860s. Frequently the symbols are inserted at a particular point of the essay, but sometimes material was added without a mark for insertion. There are also inserted notes marked for a particular page, some of which are obviously drafts of other work, published or unpublished. The symbols for such additions are noted as such by a bracketed editorial note.

Short additions in Budd's hand or interlined additions are frequently inserted in the essay itself; those are set off by a single bar, |, and conclude with a bracketed editorial note — [added], [alternate wording], etc. — after the manner of Nora Barlow's edition of Charles Darwin's ornithological notes (*Bull. Br. Museum (Nat. Hist.) Hist. Ser.,* 1963, *2,* 201–78).

The third set of notes consists of those added by the editor; they are enclosed within square brackets.

In general, the text is as written, the chief exception being that Budd's abbreviations and contractions generally conclude with the last letter written over the period — D^r, 4th etc. — while the printed version places these letters on the line before the period — Dr., 4th., etc. I have made occasional silent corrections in spelling and punctuation, but these have been kept to a minimum, and inconsistencies, such as use of *shew* and *show,* have been retained as written. In questions that result from variations in handwriting, such as the occasional capitalization of nouns in mid-sentence, I have exercised editorial judgment without comment. Long quotations have been set as extracts for clarity. Material in braces, { }, has been scratched out in the manuscript. Material in brackets, [ ], is editorial. Material in brackets within quotations is sometimes Budd's editorial additions, which have been indicated in the appropriate note; all other editorial additions are mine. Where Budd had altered a quotation, the correct wording is frequently provided in brackets following *sic.* Large sections of the manuscript in chapters one or two have been marked "quote" or "Q." Budd used some of the marked sections in his later published papers, but not all of them. Some sections of the essay not marked for quotation also appear in later publications. Possibly Budd intended marks for his 1842 revisions or his 1843 Bristol paper, but it has been impossible to determine their actual purpose. They have *not* been indicated in the printed text. The only other routine omission has been underlining for emphasis added in pencil; these emphases have been omitted to present the essay, as closely as possible, in its original form.

ACKNOWLEDGMENTS

The editor gratefully acknowledges the permission of the National Library of Medicine, owner of the manuscript, and Mrs. Richard Harper, widow of the greatgrandson of William Budd's brother Richard, to publish the essay. Quotations from Budd's letters are by courtesy of the Wellcome Trustees. This publication was supported in part by NIH grant LM 03245 from the National Library of Medicine. The editor's original interest in the work of William Budd was the result of research begun in the seminar of Professor Josef Altholz. The work could not have been completed without the cooperation and assistance of many individuals. In particular: Mr. Eric Freeman, librarian of the Wellcome Institute, and Dr. Manfred Waserman, curator of modern manuscripts, History of Medicine Division, National Library of Medicine gave invaluable help; Drs. Kenneth Keele and William Bynum arranged for the editor's admission to several London libraries; Professor Stanford Lehmberg provided an introduction to the Institute of Historical Research; Mr. Alexander M. Rodger, librarian, Royal College of Physicians and Surgeons at Glasgow, was particularly helpful in tracing the ideas of the Glasgow physicians; and the staffs of several libraries, including the University of Minnesota, the London School of Hygiene and Tropical Medicine, the British Museum, the Wellcome Institute, the National Library of Medicine, and the Royal Society of Medicine, were also very helpful. While in England, the editor was made welcome by Mrs. Harper and her sons, Drs. Peter and John Harper, and learned much from them about the history of the Budd family. Mrs. Ann Adams kindly shared knowledge collected for a family biography. The secretaries of the Department of History of Medicine, University of Minnesota, Ms. Katherine Kosiak and Mr. David Wood, have typed a number of drafts. Professor Leonard Wilson repeatedly read the material and provided valuable historical and editorial suggestions that greatly improved the final product. Dr. John Blake of the National Library of Medicine read the typescript and provided helpful suggestions. All remaining defects and limitations are the sole responsibility of the editor.

INTRODUCTION:

TYPHOID FEVER RESEARCH AND THE ORIGIN OF WILLIAM BUDD'S THACKERAY PRIZE ESSAY

The average person's life expectancy increased during the Victorian era, apparently because of declining death rates and especially the reduction in the proportion of deaths due to infectious diseases. Most infectious diseases had once been classified as fevers, although by Victorian times many had been identified as specific diseases; yet confusion remained. The infectious disease that served the medical profession as a model during this period was typhoid, or enteric, fever.[1]

Charles Creighton's *History of Epidemics in Britain* discussed the continued fevers and noted that it was not until 1869 that enteric fever deaths were tabulated separately by the registrar-general.[2] He commented that "deaths from enteric fever . . . remained somewhat steady (in a growing population) for about ten years after the separation, and then began to decline."[3] Royston Lambert, in his biography of Sir John Simon, also noted a decline in fever cases at approximately the same period.[4] While the exact timing varied, the same pattern was seen in other western countries.[5]

The degree to which various reforms were important in this decline of typhoid fever as a major health problem can probably never be determined. Of greatest importance was the general awareness of the value of hygiene — both public and personal — which increased steadily from the early Victorian period of sanitary reform. Another important factor may have been a better-nourished population, which was better able to withstand the attack of fever. There is no solid evidence for such a hypothesis, but a general improvement in the standard of living makes it probable. Somewhere among the general improvement, a place should be made for an increased knowledge of typhoid fever and the effects of this knowledge on the practice of private physicians and public medical officers.

It was only in the twentieth century that typhoid fever was brought under control, for, while the general improvement in sewerage and the efforts to provide pure water lowered morbidity and mortality in the nineteenth century, serious problems remained, and typhoid fever epidemics continued to occur despite precautions. Actual control was possible only after the isolation of the bacterial cause of the disease. The identification of carriers, the recognition of the role of shellfish in the spread of the disease, and the proper training of experts in public health and sanitary engineering — all required bacteriology.[6]

The search for and discovery of the typhoid bacillus in the 1880s was the result of the maturation of the germ theory but also required that physicians recognize specific diseases that would have specific causes. The recognition of typhoid fever as a specific disease was the result of careful research by a generation of physicians. Even after the specificity was conceded, questions remained about the nature of its cause and the means of its propagation. A leader in the campaign to establish that it was due to a specific material cause and that it was "essentially contagious," a new case always resulting from a previous one, was William Budd of Bristol, England.[7] His medical career spanned the period when the specificity of typhoid fever was established. He was a student when Pierre Louis first published his work on typhoid, and he died in 1880, the year Carl Eberth identified the typhoid bacillus. Budd's work and its reception, therefore, reflect the growing understanding of typhoid fever in the Victorian period, an understanding that made possible the eventual control of the disease.

In 1840 William Budd submitted an unsuccessful essay for the Thackeray Prize of the Provincial Medical and Surgical Association, and he mentioned it in a footnote to his classic 1859 paper on the contagiousness of typhoid fever.[8] E. W. Goodall and Margaret Pelling have reconstructed Budd's thoughts on typhoid circa 1840 by reference to his published statements on the essay and his extant letters, but both assumed that the original essay was lost because it was not in any known collection of Budd papers.[9] In the National Library of Medicine (NLM), Bethesda, Maryland, there is an anonymous essay manuscript that is without doubt a Thackeray Prize essay and that, on the basis of internal evidence, must be William Budd's contribution.[10]

The Thackeray Prize was the earliest scientific award given by the Provincial Medical and Surgical Association (forerunner of the British Medical Association), and, while it was awarded only once, it is referred to in the various historical accounts of the association.[11] The association desired to encourage scientific research, but it was struggling to exist from year to year. The prize was not an institutional success, but its evolution and results were carefully recorded in the minutes of the young association.

During the first year of its existence the Provincial Medical and Surgical Association began to consider the propriety of establishing an annual monetary prize for the best essay on a medical or surgical subject. Its council did not believe it wise to commit any portion of the annual dues income to such a prize but was pleased to receive from a council member, Dr. William M. Thackeray of Chester, the suggestion that a special endowment fund be raised to support it. Dr. Thackeray gave five pounds to the treasury on condition that, "If nineteen other individuals would subscribe twenty pounds each, and place the money in some public security, [he] would add fifteen more to the sum [he] ha[d] transmitted. The interest of the £400 might be given annually for the best Essay on some Medical or Surgical subject."[12] At the annual meeting the members decided to open a subscription fund to enable the association to grant such prizes; the fund was to accumulate until it totaled five hundred pounds, after which its annual interest yield would be used for essay prizes.[13]

The fund grew very slowly; in 1834 the council reported a total of three donors and forty pounds.[14] No other contributions were obtained until 1837, when Dr. Thackeray increased his contribution to fifty pounds, to be given as a prize on a subject selected by the council. Dr. Thackeray's only condition was that the competition be open to all regular medical practitioners of the United Kingdom.[15] The council approved the idea of a prize, to be called the Thackeray Prize, and recommended that the subject be determined at the annual meeting at Cheltenham and the essays submitted in June 1838.[16] At the meeting a committee consisting of "Dr. Barlow, Mr. Crosse, Dr. John Conolly, Dr. Lyon, Mr. Hetling, Mr. Soden, and Dr. Forbes" was appointed to select a subject. It could not agree on a subject and asked for two months to deliberate. It also suggested the essays be submitted by 1 May 1839.[17]

The prize competition was announced publicly in December 1837; essays were to be submitted by 1 January 1840, and the subject was "the investigation of the sources of the common Continued Fevers of Great Britain and Ireland, and the ascertaining of the circumstances which favour the diffusion of these diseases; and also those circumstances which may have a tendency to render them communicable from one person to another."[18]

At the meeting held in July 1838, the council informed the association of the announcement and recommended the appointment of a committee of judges. The president, vice presidents (all past presidents were permanent vice presidents of the association), Drs. Forbes and Conolly were selected as the adjudication committee.[19]

At the annual meeting in July 1840, Dr. Forbes announced that
eight essays had been submitted and that all had been read by Drs.
Jeffreys (the president) and Conolly and himself. The judges recommended the essay written by Dr. William Davidson, senior physician of
the Glasgow Royal Infirmary, and the association so awarded the
Thackeray Prize.[20]

Three other essays received honorable mention. One, "bearing the
motto from Howard 'If it were asked what is the cause of gaol fever,'
&c.," was judged "not equal in all respects" to the winning essay but was
"a very valuable memoir." This is the NLM manuscript. It was clearly
favored over the other two that received notice, each of which was said to
contain "many valuable facts and observations."[21] Dr. Davidson's essay
was printed and the others were presumably returned to their authors.[22]
Dr. Budd, at least, seems to have had his essay in his possession when he
wrote his 1859 paper.

The topic chosen by the association, the continued fevers of Great
Britain, was hardly surprising; the questions surrounding the concept of
fever were among the most important in early Victorian medicine. Most
provincial practitioners were observing febrile diseases in their practices
and many hoped to make some contribution to the solution of the problem. George Eliot captures this concern brilliantly in her character Ter-
tius Lydgate, the provincial surgeon of Middlemarch. Mr. Lydgate's
training at Paris, Edinburgh, and London, and his professional aspira-
tion — to establish a research hospital for the study of "fever or fevers"
and to enlighten the scientific world concerning the remaining "dark ter-
ritories of Pathology" — were strikingly paralleled in William Budd and
many other provincial practitioners.[23]

The questions surrounding the concept of fever, which were as old as
rational medicine, had become particularly acute in the early nineteenth
century. The development of medical sciences and the study of disease in
hospitals made possible greater precision and more accurate criticism.
Equally important, the growth of cities as a result of the industrial
revolution was accompanied by a great increase in the frequency of
fevers. In addition to the usual epidemics, fever became endemic in
some localities, particularly among the working classes and especially in
times of economic distress.

The members of the Provincial Medical and Surgical Association
were keenly interested in the nature, causes, and propagation of continued fever because such fevers played an extremely large role in their
practices. The central question, only rarely addressed because Victorian

physicians knew their answers were at best incomplete, was, Is fever a disease or a symptom of disease? The answer was never simple because so much seemed to depend on the particulars of any individual case. A more promising and pragmatically more important question was, How can fever be prevented? By 1838 several young physicians, influenced by the utilitarian philosophy of Jeremy Bentham, had begun to investigate the role of fever in the public health, particularly its relationship to poverty and disease among the kingdom's poor.[24] The frequent occurrence of fever among the poor, especially in times of scarcity and trade depression, was well known, but the relationship was not simply one of cause and effect. During the period of trade depression following the Napoleonic Wars, a consensus concerning fever had emerged based largely on the epidemic experience and the medical theories of the eighteenth century. William Budd initially shared in this consensus.

Budd was born 14 September 1811 at North Tawton, Devon, the fourth son and sixth child of Samuel Budd, a surgeon, and his wife, Catherine Wreford Budd. Both parents were well educated, and Mr. Budd had seen service as a naval surgeon in the war with France during 1794. The family was sufficiently well-to-do that all nine sons received university educations, six in medicine.[25]

William Budd's early education occurred at home; his younger brothers had tutors, and Catherine Budd recalled late in life that the elder children tutored the younger ones. His medical education was not unusual; while the Apothecaries Act of 1815 had begun the reform of medical education, there were still numerous formats for one wishing to qualify. The typical means was apprenticeship to a medical practitioner, frequently a surgeon-apothecary, supplemented by observation of the practice at some hospital. William Budd began his studies with his father and may have read the works of the great naval surgeons of the eighteenth century — James Lind, Gilbert Blane, and Thomas Trotter — with which he was clearly familiar later in his career. His early knowledge of fever was the result of his father's teaching and experience. It no doubt included some familiarity with the fever experience of the postwar epidemics.

The terms of fever study used in the early nineteenth century had been established by the great Dutch medical teacher, Herman Boerhaave, who had, early in the eighteenth century, achieved a productive blend of theoretical explanations, based on the best contemporary science, and of clinical observation, especially of particular epidemics and the conditions associated with them. The parameters of the explanation had been modified in the course of the century by the development of neural pathology, but the essential balance of theory and observation had been preserved. In the late eighteenth century, William Cullen, an Edinburgh medical professor, modified the explanation of fevers in light of what he thought was the real, clinically observed, absence of inflammation and presence of debility in patients suffering from fever.

Cullen's concept of typhus had been modified by the experiences of British physicians, particularly naval physicians, serving in other parts of the world. Following the lead of John Pringle, an army surgeon, James Lind, Sir Gilbert Blane, and Thomas Trotter published influential studies of the role of fevers in naval medicine. These physicians were closely associated with domestic practitioners who often had colonial experience and who led the fever hospital movement, establishing special wards or institutions devoted to the isolation of fever patients and the study of fever. Among the most influential writers of this group were John Haygarth of Chester, James Currie of Liverpool, John Clark of Newcastle, and Robert Willan of London.[26] By the time of Cullen's death in 1790, the leading British fever theorists saw all fever as interrelated; it was associated with lack of proper hygiene and other environmental factors, although it could become contagious. Fever was generally viewed as debilitating, and, therefore, to be treated by stimulants such as Peruvian bark and wine.

This consensus dominated the observations of the post–Napoleonic War fever epidemics, and the studies of them by various authors in various locations were remarkably similar. Two of the most influential theorists were Thomas Bateman, physician of the London Fever Hospital, and Edward Percival, physician to the Hardwicke Fever Hospital in Dublin.[27] For both Bateman and Percival there was only one kind of continued, essential febrile disease, and both called it *typhus*. According to Percival,

> the term typhus, as a generic appellation of the family of fevers here referred to, appears to me wholly unobjectionable. It is sufficiently comprehensive in its original import; and long use, . . . has notoriously appropriated it to the class of epidemic and contagious fevers now under consideration. . . . [He suggests three divisions — Typhus gravior, T. mitior, and T. mitissimus.] Thus, the same generic term will be preserved, in three several species or grades of the same generic disease.
>
> Those who are most familiar with the aspect of epidemic fevers on a large scale, will be least disposed to separate them into distinct genera. . . . Each of these species commences with some congestive

or inflammatory diathesis; each may decline with stupor, sub-delirium and death; . . . . Neither do the mildest nor the severest species propagate merely their own forms, but rather seem to generate each other promiscuously, ...[28]

For Percival, individual cases in each species could be further characterized by an organ or organ system particularly affected or inflamed — "cephalic, pulmonic, enteric, etc."[29]

Dr. Bateman went even further, for all of his experience "tended more and more to impress [him] with the conviction of the identity of that disease under all its modifications." "The great variety of form, which fever constantly assumes in different individuals, and which has rendered its identity questionable, occasions considerable difficulties in classing its modifications or constituting distinct varieties for practical purposes." This being so, Bateman suggested that the disease be described as typhus in either a simple or complicated form, the "more complicated varieties connected with different degrees of acute and sub-acute inflammation."[30]

In an 1821 review of many of the works published since 1817 on the epidemics, the reviewer concluded: "It is gratifying to find that, in all essential points writers so highly qualified agree; . . . . All of them agree in considering continued fever as a pathological state. . . ." Typhus was the recognized term for this state that began with excitement and ended in debility. Contagion had played an important role in the spread of the fever, but cases arose spontaneously as well. Such spontaneous cases were further spread by contagion under the proper conditions — "in crowded and ill-ventilated apartments, and among the poor depressed by misery, cold and want." An early antiphlogistic treatment was generally adopted, and fever was seen as related to inflammation in some unknown or unsuspected way; it could frequently be complicated by the inflammation of particular organs.[31] But on the subject of the relationship to inflammation there was a minority opinion of some standing, and in Britain its chief spokesman was Henry Clutterbuck.[32]

An apprentice-trained surgeon who spent a year on the wards of the United Boroughs Hospital in London before he qualified as a surgeon, Clutterbuck was influenced strongly by Hunterian pathology, and the local cause of disease was a vital part of his surgical heritage.[33] Clutter-buck desired to qualify also in medicine and in 1802 attended medical lectures at Edinburgh; in 1804 he received his M.D. from Glasgow with a thesis on fever. In this work he advanced the idea "that fever, strictly so called, or what is termed idiopathic fever, is, in its origin, a local and not a general disease; and that it consists essentially in inflammation of the cerebral substance. . . ."[34] In 1807 Clutterbuck expanded his thesis and republished it; a second edition appeared in 1825. That febrile symptoms were similar to those of inflammations had long been recognized, but it was Clutterbuck's claim that inflammation occurred in the brain, different degrees and areas of affection explaining the clinical diversity, and caused a secondary debility as a result of previously occurring vascular excitement in the cerebral tissue. This combination of the pathophysiology of debility and the study of inflammation was a natural outgrowth of his training. He obviously had been influenced strongly by the ideas of William Cullen, and quite possibly by those of Cullen's students, Benjamin Rush or John Brown, but, in the Hunterian tradition, Clutterbuck had confirmed, to his own satisfaction, his clinical and theoretical doctrines in the autopsy room. It was his belief that he had consistently found evidence of cerebral inflammation in the postmortem examination of deceased fever patients.

Clutterbuck returned to London and after publication of his work became one of the most successful practitioners in the city. He was a physician to the general dispensary from 1809 and gave extramural lectures on medicine. His income from these lectures alone was said to have at one time exceeded a thousand pounds a year.[35] In 1837 he claimed that the change in therapeutic fashion, the bloodletting revolution, of the early nineteenth century was at least in part the result of the adoption of his ideas that fever was essentially secondary to inflammation, even if many practitioners did not adopt his localization of that inflammation in the brain.[36]

Clutterbuck had undertaken postmortem research to find the local inflammation that caused fever, but his research methods and analysis were primitive and perhaps influenced by the theory. He had clear cases of cerebrospinal inflammation, but he also resorted to "evidence of previously existing inflammation" when the actual death resulted from "secondary phenomena."[37] Clutterbuck's experience was early in the development of the new science of pathology, and his methods were not adequate to the task, as was recognized by many British reviewers of his work.[38] The explanation was too simple and did not conform to the realities of the fever experience. In the hospitals of Paris the new medical science was making its greatest progress, and, shortly after the end of the Napoleonic Wars in 1815 as well as during some intermissions in the conflict, English students visited the Paris hospitals, where they learned the techniques of clinical-pathological correlation and the maturing concepts of histology advanced by Xavier Bichat.

William Budd had opportunities for more than the minimal apprenticeship training, and in the autumn of 1828 he went to Paris for further
study. There he studied anatomy with Jean Cruveilhier, physiology with
André Marie Duméril, medicinal chemistry with Matthew Orfila, but
most importantly attended the lectures in physiology, pathology, and
internal medicine given by François Broussais.[39] Broussais was at the
height of his fame and influence as a teacher; his doctrine of physiological medicine was exerting a profound influence. Broussais, like Clutterbuck, attributed all fever to local inflammation but, unlike Clutterbuck,
located it in the gastrointestinal mucosa. Broussais, the son of a provincial surgeon, volunteered for service in the revolutionary wars. In 1798
he was given leave to attend the new medical school in Paris, where in
1803 he graduated, profoundly influenced by Bichat's method of tissue
analysis. Broussais returned to active military service and moved with
the armies of Napoleon throughout Europe. During this time, he tried to
continue his researches but lacked supervision and facilities. Despite
difficulties, Broussais published in 1808 a monograph on the study of
inflammations, primarily of the trunk.[40]

This work was a valiant first effort and it won praise from Philippe
Pinel and other leaders of Paris medicine. In it Broussais described his
clinical and postmortem observations on the soldiers he treated in Italy
during 1806, beginning with what was for him the paradigm case of his
fellow army surgeon Beau. Broussais performed autopsies routinely, but
his descriptions of postmortem findings were brief and often lacked
precision. In his autopsies he looked for gross changes believed to indicate sites of local inflammation. In the one-paragraph report on Beau, he
observed a contracted stomach with a thick, red mucous membrane and
assumed that Beau had died of gastritis. In other cases of soldiers dying
after acute fevers, he observed inflammation and ulcers in the intestinal
mucosa as well. Broussais advanced the hypothesis that fever was the
result of gastroenteritis. By 1816 he had developed a complete explanation of variations in symptoms based on the physiology of membranes he
had learned from Bichat.

Several factors may have conspired against Broussais in his effort to
understand fever. The theory, prevalent in military medicine particularly, that many fevers were inflammatory in nature led to severe antiphlogistic therapy. The result of such heroic therapeutic efforts could be,
according to Esmond Long, that it was difficult for the inexperienced
pathologist to distinguish the "anatomic results of the vastly overener-
getic purgings and bleedings and starvings of [then] current practice"
from the "manifestations of primary disease."[41] A second consideration

was that the realities of camp life in the Napoleonic armies were such that enteric diseases such as typhoid fever and dysentery, with their very real effect on the intestinal mucosa, were extremely prevalent. Finally, and perhaps most important, Broussais was looking for evidence of inflammation and might have easily seen the reddened, thick mucous membranes of the stomach as such when, in all probability, what he actually saw, perhaps for the first time, was a normal stomach. Frank and Ruth Mann have pointed out that if autopsies are delayed several hours, postmortem digestion will destroy much of the gastric mucous membrane. Delay can also lead to a settling of blood in the stomach wall. In the field Broussais probably performed autopsies much more promptly than would have been done in Paris hospitals or medical schools and, as a result, he would have found more of the mucosa intact, but possibly also with some reddening, suggesting the appearance of gastritis.[42] According to William Boyd, death agonies can contract the stomach, thickening the mucous membrane, and agonal vascular congestion may redden it, leading, if based on gross findings alone, to the still frequent mistaken diagnosis of gastritis in the twentieth century.[43] Such possibility of artifact was recognized in Broussais's work by René Laennec, who cautioned against equating redness with inflammation of the mucosal surfaces. "We ought . . . to be certain that the appearances presented to us have not been the result of decomposition after death or of congestions which take place, . . . especially in the last agony. . . . If these principles are disregarded . . . pathological anatomy . . . will soon . . . become a mere tissue of hypotheses, founded on optical illusions and fanciful speculations without any real benefit to medicine."[44]

Following Broussais's first expression of his ideas in 1808, there occurred in Paris, between 1811 and 1813, an epidemic of fever, and in 1813 Marc Anton Petit and Etienne R. A. Serres published a careful study of the fever cases as they were seen at the Hôtel Dieu.[45] Lesions of the lower portion of the ileum were recognized as characteristic of the particular epidemic and differentiated it, in the minds of Petit and Serres, from ordinary enteritis. They did not locate the ulcers in the glands of Peyer and Brunner, but from the color engravings in their work and the symptoms described as characterizing the illness, subsequent pathologists have generally regarded the disease as typhoid fever. In their illustrations one can clearly see their depiction of the normal intestine, the beginnings of inflammation in the glands, the beginning of ulceration, and evidence of healing with perforation during convalescence. They coordinated the course of the disease with the lesions and thought that the severity of the fever was determined by the extent of the inflammation. While Petit and Serres argued that the evidence, clinical and pathological, suggested a unique disease, Broussais coopted their results in his teachings on the ubiquitous occurrence of gastroenteritis, and the two researchers do not seem to have challenged his interpretation. Despite the reservations of a few French pathologists like Laennec, Broussais's interpretation of fever as gastroenteritis gained popularity and converts in the 1820s.

Another related effort to use pathological anatomy in the study of fevers may be seen in the 1821 work of August Chomel.[46] Where Clutterbuck and Broussais had turned to pathological anatomy to find evidence of inflammation that they knew existed, Chomel looked to pathological anatomy for evidence of secondary differences that would explain the diversity of symptoms among the essential fevers seen clinically. In 1798 Philippe Pinel had arranged the large number of clinical variants of fever described by eighteenth-century medical writers in his nosography of the essential fevers. Chomel, trained in the teachings of Pinel and Bichat at the new, postrevolution Paris medical school, viewed febrile diseases in Pinel's terms. He separated the periodic from the continued fevers, tried to define fever as a general pathological state, and then began to consider its variants. He acknowledged the intestinal lesion described by Petit and Serres as being very frequent, even present constantly for long periods in Paris hospital practice, but cases of fever did occur without them, so that he thought the lesion was only of secondary importance. Chomel attempted to synthesize all past observations and add, whenever relevant, postmortem observations. He described inflammatory fever in essentially the same terms as those used by Boerhaave over a century before; nervous fever much as George Cheyne had done in 1733; and adynamic fever, using Pinel's term for the slow fever described by John Huxham in 1750. There was for Chomel a bilious fever that was strikingly similar to that described by James Lind in 1768, and a mucous fever as seen by Broussais and Petit and Serres. Chomel failed to find gross postmortem similarities, and what pathological and anatomical findings he does record could explain the clinical diversity only partially.

In 1824 Gabriel Andral, a dynamic young physician and teacher, began to publish his increasingly popular clinical lectures. In the first edition he begins his discussion of fevers by accepting Pinel's nosography. Unlike Chomel, Andral spent relatively less time on the literature of the past and more on his own clinical observations. But, like Chomel, he still sought postmortem explanations for clinically observed variations among the essential fevers rather than treating pathological anatomy as an equal partner with clinical observation. Both Chomel and Andral were teaching in Paris in 1828, but there is no information on William Budd's knowledge of their ideas. It is known that he studied extensively with Broussais. He may also have been aware of English research on the pathology of fevers.

A greater degree of balance was achieved in England, and two significant reports appeared on a London fever epidemic of 1825–26. The first of these, published in the late summer of 1826, was by Cornwallis Hewett, physician to St. George's Hospital, London. Dr. Hewett found that during the epidemic the London fever was characterized at postmortem by "follicular ulcerations of the bowels." Hewett recognized that the lesion occurred in the glands of Peyer and related the lesions to the increased frequency of abdominal symptoms and diarrhea seen in the 1825–26 epidemic. He argued that among the causes of the epidemic there would be an explanation for what he saw as a pathological stopping-up of the orifices of the glands. The glands distended by their secretions then became disorganized. Yet for Dr. Hewett, even though the follicular ulceration was characteristic of the 1825–26 epidemic, it was only a temporary complication in the general course of idiopathic fever seen in London.[47]

The second report of the 1825–26 epidemic was by Richard Bright, physician to Guy's Hospital. Bright studied disease intensively, and his contributions are well known. In his 1827 *Reports of Medical Cases* he described the fever cases and included beautifully prepared plates to illustrate his findings. He clearly feared Broussais's and Clutterbuck's theory of fever as the result of local inflammation yet recognized the importance of his own observations.

> Whatever may be the primary nature of the febrile attack, there can be no doubt that early in the disease, not only in the season of which I have spoken, but almost always, the intestinal canal is irritated, and that this irritation keeps up all the bad symptoms. . . . The appearances which are most marked in the mucous membranes of the intestines are those of increased action, vascularity sometimes occurring in patches of greater or less extent. . . . This vascularity is more generally connected with inflammation of the mucous glands, which often appear like the small-pox on the second or third day of eruption.

Bright's illustrations show clearly that he, like Petit and Serres, was seeing typhoid fever and that he understood clearly that the disease was in some way related to the characteristic lesion of the small bowel. He acknowledged further that, while in individual cases other organs might suffer more or less extensively than the intestines, "there is decidedly no class of morbid appearances so frequent, and none more important, than those which involve the structure of the intestines. . . ."[48] Yet Bright, while recognizing the importance of the lesion, had to acknowledge that its frequency was *almost* always, that there were other lesions, that he did not understand the primary nature of fever, but that these intestinal lesions would not explain it satisfactorily.

Respect for the evidence of the postmortem room might lead to greater understanding, but the clinical nature of fever remained so nebulous that equality of postmortem and clinical evidence could not resolve the questions. To claim a position of superiority for postmortem findings was both difficult and dangerous — difficult because clinical data about a living patient seemed much more closely related to medical practice, and dangerous because of the great potential for excess. As Bright had observed, the lesions of the bowel and the inflammation associated with them were insufficient to explain fever as a general state; to attempt to do so was to return to the fallacies of Clutterbuck and Broussais.

In the 1820s two French physicians were able to establish the primacy of postmortem data, yet to avoid making the idiopathic fever simply the result of a local inflammation. In the process they defined typhoid fever as a specific disease entity. The first to do so was Pierre Bretonneau, physician to the general hospital at Tours.

As an officer of health in country practice, Bretonneau experienced rural epidemics of fever in 1802 and again in 1812. Rural epidemics tend to be particularly well defined medical events because one practitioner often sees all the cases and can form a clear clinical picture of the disease. Epidemics were responsible for most of the clear clinical distinctions of the eighteenth century, and the importance of rural epidemics of typhoid fever has been clearly illustrated by the experience of the New England physician Nathan Smith, whose essay on typhous fever has been cited repeatedly by subsequent writers for clarity and modernity. In the epidemics of 1802 and 1812 Bretonneau achieved a clear clinical picture of a particular fever, which he recognized again in 1819 when an epidemic of fever broke out at Tours. Under rural conditions each person was usually subject to the disease only once, and the clearly contagious

course of the epidemic as it spread from person to person strongly suggested the spread of a single specific disease. As a student of Bichat and
Corvisart, Bretonneau wished to study the pathological anatomy of disease; in 1819, as a hospital physician, he finally had an opportunity to do
so. As a result of his rural experience, Bretonneau could diagnose the
epidemic fever cases in Tours clearly, and at postmortem, in these cases,
he invariably found smallpoxlike pustules in the lining of the intestine.
He stressed the need to compare the postmortem anatomy of fever
patients with normal anatomy and with other cases of acute disease and
performed over 300 autopsies on humans and animals. He performed
120 autopsies on cases of fever, clearly locating the lesion on the intestinal glands and distinguishing it from tubercular ulceration, dysentery,
erythema of the gastrointestinal mucosa, and postmortem artifacts.
Bretonneau carefully described the course of the disease, observing that
its severity was unrelated to the number or extent of the ulcerations of
the bowel. He named the disease *dothienenteritis* — boils or pox of the intestine — based on the constant occurrence of the ulcerations in the small
intestine.[49] It is difficult to say with certainty whether the idea of specificity of disease based on autopsy findings, the "ontology" of Corvisart and
Laennec, or the experience of specific epidemics in rural settings was the
initial key to Bretonneau's understanding — ideas and experience constantly and reciprocally influenced each other through the 1820s. In his
funeral oration for the Tours physician, Bretonneau's pupil Armand
Trousseau laid primary emphasis on Bretonneau's disease experience.[50]

In 1824 Trousseau was Bretonneau's intern when he was powerfully
impressed by the clarity of the concept of dothienenteritis. On his return
to Paris, Trousseau discovered that his master's unpublished ideas were
not secure. In 1826 Trousseau wrote, "I wish to give a sketch of his
labors in order to call the attention of physicians to a disease extremely
frequent, but hardly studied until the present, and also to ensure Dr.
Bretonneau the possession of his discovery which they have already
wished to take from him."[51] Just who "they" were is not clear in the text,
but one can easily imagine that it may have been Pierre Louis, who was
working along similar lines at La Charité Hospital in Paris. However,
Trousseau may also have had in mind any of several recently published
researches on the pathology of fevers or the pathological anatomy of the
gastrointestinal mucosa that he cited in the article.[52] He compared the
partially developed observations of such writers to twelve cases from
Bretonneau's clinic in Tours, five with autopsies, and outlined briefly
Bretonneau's ideas on the specificity of the intestinal inflammation and

the contagious nature of the disease. He called attention to the fact that Bretonneau's students, beginning with Velpeau in 1820, had been discussing these ideas in the Paris hospitals and that the investigations of disease of the 1820s must be considered in the light of such discussions.

Probably any work on fever in the Paris hospitals during the 1820s was influenced in some degree by informal discussion, but one should not assign too great a role to it. Bretonneau's experience was based on a particular epidemic and on his unique ability to diagnose the epidemic fever as a result of his experience with the same disease in the countryside. Parisian physicians, with larger experience, could readily accept that Bretonneau had observed lesions in the small bowel in all cases of the 1819 epidemic at Tours without accepting the belief that such lesions defined a specific febrile disease. As long as the accumulated experience of physicians was viewed as equal in validity to observations on a single epidemic, it was virtually impossible to bring order out of the chaos.[53]

The experience of Pierre Louis was critical, therefore, because he successfully abandoned the past. Trained at Paris, Louis had gone to Russia to practice, but, disillusioned by his inability to help patients, he returned to Paris in 1820 to study medicine in the wards and deadhouse of La Charité. Among the new techniques of medicine in the French capital of 1820 was mediate auscultation, and Louis, interested in new methods of medicine, may have studied auscultation with Laennec. One of Laennec's controversial claims was that tubercles were always present in cases of phthisis. Louis personally investigated this claim and became an acknowledged master of the study of pulmonary disease. As a researcher he extended the methods developed by the early pathologists in that he not only kept detailed clinical and postmortem case records, but also recorded detailed descriptions of the appearance of *all* major organs and tissues when *he* performed an autopsy. He then carefully tabulated such records so that he could state the exact number of patients who had exhibited a particular symptom or lesion and could correlate the two with a numerical precision never before attempted. This admittedly crude statistical approach, the famous numerical method, enabled Louis to confirm Laennec's idea of the unitary nature of phthisis.[54] Louis's numerical method also enabled him to appreciate the importance of a universally occurring postmortem observation in the definition of disease.

The emerging concept of specificity of disease as defined by constantly occurring anatomical lesions slowly gained ground among a small number of anatomic pathologists in the 1820s. The work and

teaching of Corvisart and the example of Laennec were of unques-
tionable importance; Broussais's attacks on the ontologists were efforts to
combat a real enemy. In 1821 Bretonneau communicated to the Acad-
émie Royale de Médecine his ideas on the specificity of diphtheria, and
they were apparently well received; in 1824 he was elected a correspond-
ing member of the academy. Also in 1824 Pierre Louis published one of
his early papers on croup, quite possibly influenced by Bretonneau's
work, which is mentioned in the article.[55]

The influence of external ideas on fever in the development of
Louis's thought is suggested by his 1823 study of perforation of the small
intestine. He reported ten cases seen in 1822 in which patients died of
perforation of the small bowel; in all, the perforation occurred in the
lower portion of the ileum. The intestinal mucous membrane was generally inflamed in varying degrees and to various depths. The patients
were all young, in good health, and newly arrived in Paris. Nine of the
cases began as a mild continued fever, with some diarrhea, but no particularly severe symptoms until the intestine was perforated. The perforation was indicated by sudden severe pain, symptoms of peritonitis, and
rapid death (after 20 to 54 hours). Louis discussed the difficulties of diagnosing the condition prior to perforation, there being no pathognomic
symptoms.[56] Louis may have begun to recognize the intestinal lesions as
a pathognomic sign after learning of Bretonneau's work, or it may have
been an independent conclusion after further research. In addition, the
patients were occasionally delirious, a symptom that further obscured
the diagnosis.

In 1829, while William Budd was studying in Paris, Louis published
his two-volume classic, *Recherches anatomiques, pathologiques et thérapeutiques
sur la maladie connue sous le nom de gastro-entérite, fièvre putride, adynamique,
ataxique, typhoide, etc.* According to Louis's own statement, he collected
observations on fever for five years, 1822–27, analyzed the records
according to the numerical method, and described the typhuslike fever
or typhoid affection of Paris hospitals. The disease was characterized by
abdominal symptoms and rose-colored lenticular spots in life and by the
constant presence of lesions of the Peyer's patches of the small intestine at
postmortem.[57] Louis defined the fever by the postmortem lesion, and the
unique distribution of idiopathic fever in Paris of the 1820s made possible the definition. There seems to have been no louse-borne typhus in
Paris at that period.

We have no information on William Budd's reaction, if any, to the
publication of Louis's treatise. His teacher, Broussais, would have con-
demned the ontological tendencies of Louis's work while claiming the

results as a confirmation of the universal presence of inflammation of the gastrointestinal mucosa in a febrile disease. Pierre Louis certainly did not wish to be linked with Broussais's teaching but thought that he was contributing to a tradition of medical investigation even more familiar to young Budd, namely, to British studies of typhus fever. In 1829 Budd became seriously ill with fever that he later believed to have been typhoid fever, and returned to North Tawton for a protracted convalescence.

The Revolution of 1830 and the cholera epidemic presumably delayed Budd's return to Paris until the summer or early fall of 1833. While studying medicine under his father, a country surgeon, he would have become familiar with the many British works on typhus fever. Budd's older brothers, who had recently begun to study medicine at Edinburgh, would probably have acquainted their father and younger brother with the newest ideas and latest research on fever.[58] In the late 1820s the leaders of British fever research were William P. Alison, professor of the institutes of medicine at Edinburgh, and Alexander Tweedie, physician to the London Fever Hospital.

William Pulteney Alison possessed extensive experience with fever epidemics, and his ideas were typical of British physicians. Serious questions had arisen about the contagiousness of endemic typhus fever; many physicians believed with John Armstrong that typhus originated in peculiar conditions of the atmosphere that permitted the generation of fever poison in the filth of crowded humanity. The poison would be produced in large quantities in particular areas, creating the impression that the fever was contagious when, in fact, it resulted from simultaneous exposure of numbers of people to the same poison. British physicians also thought that, once fever had been generated in this way, the bodies of those ill with it produced and gave off into the air further poison.[59] In 1815 William Alison, aged twenty-five, was a newly appointed physician to the New Town Dispensary in Edinburgh, and his experience of fever epidemics during several years after 1815 left an indelible impression on his mind.[60]

Alison, with many of his counterparts throughout Britain, noted that while the fever epidemic was severe among the poor, who lived in crowded and dirty habitations, it was not restricted to areas of poor hygiene. As the epidemic progressed, he came to realize that, while the filth was proportioned fairly evenly among sections inhabited by the poor, the fever was confined to particular localities. Finally, he found that isolation of early cases in a particular area could halt the spread of the disease.[61]

In the press of the epidemic Dr. Alison paid little attention to clinical

variations among fever cases, although he realized that symptoms differed among different patients and that some cases were more severe
than others.[62] In 1820 Alison became a professor in the Edinburgh
medical school, where he used his experience with the endemic fevers of
that city in his clinical teaching and drew the attention of students to the
clinical variations presented by fever patients. When, in 1826-27, a
fever epidemic again broke out at Edinburgh, his analysis was clearer.

Alison still stressed the contagious nature of the fever, citing strong
arguments against a miasmatic cause of the epidemic. The disease
occurred at some times in houses that were at all other times healthy, the
only difference being the presence of fever patients, who could communicate the disease to others. Fever occurred in all sections of the city
under all varieties of conditions, and when it once entered a house or
group of houses, it broke out in rapid succession among the inhabitants.
The fever spread at a rate proportionate to the closeness of the contact of
the healthy with the sick. Finally, the disease could be observed in particular cases to be imported into a previously healthy district by persons
known to be ill or to have been exposed to one who was ill with the fever,
while the removal and isolation of the ill would halt the spread of the
disease.[63]

Dr. Alison was most interested in establishing the contagious nature
of the fever of Edinburgh because prompt isolation of fever patients
could then be used to control epidemics, but he also studied the nature of
the disease process and its complications. He viewed typhus as an
asthenia in which the chief danger, in simple or uncomplicated cases,
was the result of "the general depressed state of the circulation."
However, the simple pathology of typhus might be complicated by local
affections or inflammations, of which he recognized three — cerebral,
respiratory, and abdominal.

Such complications, while having real pathological evidences and
symptomatic differences, were subtle clinical differentiations. Dr. Alison
presented the statistics of the epidemic in which the majority of simple
cases and the mortality and frequency of the various complications were
documented. But he cautioned, "No numerical statement of this kind
can give all the information which it is desirable to convey regarding the
circumstances of the fatal cases. In almost all these, more or less complications of the general symptoms of fever with local affections not
essential to the fever is observed, but it seldom happens that the degree
of this local affection is such that it can fairly be regarded as the sole
cause of death."[64] Alison was clearly warning against the simplistic local

pathology of Clutterbuck and Broussais; in the 1820s the study of fever in Scotland remained essentially clinical.

Symptoms indicative of cerebral involvement were "urgent headache at first, and then the more active delirium, tremors, spasms, [and] coma." In the complication of the respiratory organs, the symptoms were a difficulty in breathing similar to that in bronchitis or pneumonia, while in those cases that were believed to have abdominal complications, Dr. Alison expected to observe "diarrhoea, with pain of abdomen."[65] In 1826–27 cerebral complications had been most common in Edinburgh, the abdominal most rare; he believed the relationship to be generally true of Britain.

Alison observed that fever behaved differently in France, where Andral had noted "that there are few cases of fever in the hospitals of Paris in which a spontaneous diarrhoea does not occur. . . ." This difference was, Alison believed, reflected in the postmortem experience of fever researchers in the two countries — the French frequently observing inflammation and ulceration of the intestinal mucosa, while Alison found it in only one of twenty-two patients autopsied at Edinburgh.[66]

In 1815 Alexander Tweedie received his M.D. degree from Edinburgh and in 1822 was named one of the physicians of the London Fever Hospital. Trained in the same school as William Alison and sharing the same experience of the postwar fever epidemics, Tweedie had very similar ideas on fever. In 1831 he described more fully the possible causes of fever. While acknowledging the importance of contagion and the obvious role of poverty, he reserved a large role for the epidemic constitution or seasonal and atmospheric conditions, impure or poorly ventilated air, and malaria or exhalations from decomposing organic matter, the last two the result of local conditions.

Tweedie did not define fever rigorously but held that any strictly unitary explanation of fever pathology was unacceptable. "There is not one, but several, organs affected; the affection, in the first instance at least, is functional. . . ." The functional derangement began in the brain and nervous system, passed on to the circulation and thence to affect any variety of organs, tissues, and systems. "When once the torch is lighted, when the circulation is quickened, and the blood consequently impelled with greater velocity through organs whose functions are already disordered, the transition from excitement to inflammation is often rapid." Predisposition, the period of the fever, the intensity of the attack, and a variety of other individual circumstances determined the future course of the disease. Inflammation could and frequently did supervene in febrile disease, but fever was not to be confused with inflammation. It was "primarily a general disease, which, however, in by far the largest proportion of cases becomes, in its progress, complicated with some local inflammation."[67]

Fever in general existed in three forms or divisions: "the continued, periodical, and eruptive, each of which may be again subdivided. . . ." Tweedie was interested in, and saw in the Fever Hospital, primarily continued forms of fever, which he subdivided as simple, complicated, and typhus. The simple fever was the basic general disease or functional derangement — "fever without evident symptoms of local inflammation." Approximately 20 percent of the cases seen at the London Fever Hospital were described as simple fever. Complicated fever was an attack of disease in which local symptoms indicated complications "in one or other of the organs of the head, chest, or belly. . . ." Complications might be confirmed by inflammation observed at autopsy but were indicated by symptoms occurring during the clinical course of the disease because the functional change might not extend to actual inflammation, though it usually did, particularly in fatal cases. Cerebral affection was "indicated by one or more of the following symptoms, pain, giddiness, sense of weight or fulness, watchfulness, and, in the advanced stages, delirium, coma, spasms, or more rarely convulsions." The respiratory complications included symptoms of croup, bronchitis, pneumonia, and pleurisy. It was important to differentiate between general fever complicated by respiratory symptoms and primary disease of the respiratory organs with symptomatic fever. Tweedie noted, "The application of the stethoscope is, in such cases, the only sure method of detecting the state of the lungs. . . . It is to be regretted, that a knowledge of its distinctive sounds is not more easily attained."[68] Finally, there could be abdominal affections complicating fever. These were indicated by pain or functional derangements of the digestive organs.

Typhus was differentiated from simple and complicated continued fever by the intensity of the attack. Tweedie defined it as "those more severe forms, in which, from the commencement, there is more considerable disturbance in the brain and nervous system, great prostration of the muscular power, with affection of the mucous membranes, and not infrequently of the cutaneous and glandular systems."[69] Typhus could exist in a simple or uncomplicated form but "it is not very common in Britain. . . ." Like other continued fevers, "it very often, in its progress, becomes complicated with some local congestion or inflammation, either in the brain, chest, or belly." Tweedie regarded "affection of the bronchial and intestinal mucous membranes as essential constituents of typhus fever," but either could become more severely affected and so result in the classification of the particular case as a case of either a respiratory or abdominal complication.

In discussing the abdominal complications of typhus and in particular the affection of the intestinal mucous membrane, Tweedie commented on the work of the French pathological anatomists. After a brief but fair statement of Broussais's experience and ideas, he noted:

> Did we find this membrane so universally inflamed as has been affirmed, this theory would have probably a better chance of being generally adopted than any which the localists have yet proposed; but when we recollect how many cases of pure fever have been examined by good anatomists, in this and other countries, and even in the very place from which the notion first emanated, and no unhealthy appearance discovered, I confess I am inclined to regard this condition of the mucous membrane, as one of the many complications of this inscrutable disease.[70]

The difference to be accounted for in comparing French experience with the British consisted in the frequency of a complication that was considered to depend on a variety of possible modifying facts.

> Though affections of the bowels are very often observed in the fevers of Britain, especially in certain epidemics, and at particular seasons, yet from the statements of Broussais, Andral, Louis, and many other continental writers, gastric irritation is more uniformly met with in the fevers of France than in this country; from which it may be inferred, that there is in this respect some peculiarity, which may possibly depend on the specific action of the febrile poison on the mucous membrane of the bowels.[71]

The coupling of the names of Pierre Louis and François Broussais by Alexander Tweedie in 1831 was no accident, for Louis's work was seen by many medical men as confirming that of Broussais, and Broussais claimed it as such. Many physicians thought that Louis shared Broussais's fault of generalization based on too limited an experience. Both Auguste Chomel and Gabriel Andral had described cases of what they believed were essential fevers without intestinal lesions. However, the confusion began to be resolved quickly; working on Chomel's wards at La Charité, Louis taught his friend to recognize typhoid fever, and in his clinical lectures published in 1834 Chomel began to discuss typhoid

fever at length.[72] In November 1829 Louis was appointed physician to
La Pitié Hospital, where he shared wards with Andral, who, under
Louis's guidance, learned to diagnose typhoid fever. The ability of
Louis, Chomel, and Andral to diagnose it made typhoid fever generally
familiar among the younger medical teachers of Paris in the early
1830s.[73]

During 1833–34, William Budd returned to Paris, his longest stay in
France; he studied zoology with Etienne Geoffroy Saint-Hilaire at the
Museum of Natural History, and botany and vegetable physiology with
Charles François Brisseau de Mirbel at the Faculty of Science of the Collège de France. He attended the pathology lectures of Gabriel Andral
and did practical dissection with Despine. He attended the clinical lectures of Jacques Lisfranc on surgery, Laurent Theodore Biet on skin
disease, and Philippe Ricord on venereal disease. He again studied
clinical medicine and pathology with Broussais but also attended the
clinics of a dynamic new teacher, Pierre Louis. William Budd, attending
the clinics of these two French physicians, was presented with a clear
choice on the most important methodological question of the day — the
role of pathological anatomy in medicine and the means of achieving
accuracy in medical research. While Budd was at Paris, the differences
between Louis and Broussais became public. In March 1834 Broussais
published the fourth volume of the third edition of his *Examen des doctrines
médicales*. In it he presented his case for physiological medicine and
attacked the use of ontological disease concepts. In 1816 he had criticized
Pinel's ideas of 1798 as ontological constructs. Pinel's nosography was
somewhat out of date in 1816 and the philosophical constructs of the
eighteenth century were easy to criticize, but the ease of Broussais's vic-
tory in 1816 was deceptive — there were few alternatives available to the
general practitioners. In 1821 in a second edition of the *Examen*,
Broussais expanded his attack to include the new anatomic pathology of
Laennec. In the third, vastly expanded edition, he criticized likewise the
work of Louis on phthisis and typhoid fever. He charged that Louis, like
Laennec and other anatomic pathologists, had selected cases to prove a
connection between the occurrence of particular symptoms and lesions
that Broussais did not believe existed. He also argued that, by failing to
relate the symptoms and lesions as cause and effect, Louis contributed to
therapeutic skepticism and did not help practitioners or patients. Nevertheless, with the exception of a few carelessly cited observations,
Broussais did not offer any clinical evidence to refute Louis's claims.
Later in 1834, in his *Examen de l'examen de M. Broussais,* Louis responded

to Broussais, carefully criticizing his use of clinical and pathological evidence and effectively defending the numerical method as the best road to further medical knowledge.[74]

Budd adopted the limited but precise methods of Pierre Louis. He may have done so as a result of chance. In a letter written from Paris on 6 December 1833 Budd described his study — "I attend the Pitié and Lisfranc exclusively" — and told of a new friend "who will be a treasure to me" — perhaps for the guidance offered to the various clinics. The new friend was "from Philadelphia, a frank open, fine young fellow."[75] It may have been through his American friend that Budd learned of Louis's clinic at La Pitié, for the Americans had then recently discovered Louis. During the four years, from 1829 to 1833, of William Budd's absence from Paris, Pierre Louis had emerged as a leading teacher of foreign students and preeminent at Paris as an anatomic pathologist and clinical investigator. That Louis's ability would be recognized first by foreign students was almost preordained by the nature of French medical education. The curriculum of the Ecole de Médecine consisted of required lectures by the members of the faculty and additional, nonmandatory lectures by other Paris hospital clinicians. La Pitié was quite far from the *école,* and the French medical students did not have time to attend the lectures of a little-known clinician at great distance from the center of their activities. After Louis moved to the Hôtel Dieu in 1837, his clinics became very popular with French medical students. Foreign students, many of them already qualified in medicine in their own countries, were not bound by the regulations of the Paris medical faculty, and, while attending the famous and required clinics, also sought out less crowded clinical centers.[76]

Crucial to the emerging understanding of fevers was the early recognition of Louis's ability by three young Americans: James Jackson, Jr., Caspar W. Pennock, and William Wood Gerhard. At the suggestion of his cousin, Charles T. Jackson, James Jackson, Jr. had sought out Louis's clinic in the fall of 1831, shortly after his arrival at Paris. Gerhard and Pennock, friends from Philadelphia, met Jackson in Paris and were guided by him toward the clinics at La Pitié. In the winter of 1832 the three Americans arranged for private tutoring by Louis, and in March Jackson and Gerhard were among the fifteen students of Louis who founded the *Société d'Observation Médicale,* designed for mutual discussion and criticism of their efforts in the hospital.[77]

James Jackson, Jr. had gone to Paris with particular goals, one of which was to investigate fever, and under Louis's tutelage he and his

companions learned to recognize clinically the continued fever of Paris
and the constant presence of lesions in the Peyer's patches if a case went
to autopsy. They learned to study disease by the numerical method and
were instilled with a desire to continue their researches. When he
returned home in the fall of 1833, James Jackson, Jr. set out to determine whether or not the continued fever of Boston was identical to
Louis's typhoid affection. With the help of his father, and of his cousin,
J. B. S. Jackson, pathologist at the Massachusetts General Hospital,
James Jackson, Jr. was able to confirm the identity, both clinically and
pathologically, of continued fever in Paris and Boston, but his results
were published posthumously, for he died following an attack of fever on
27 March 1834.[78]

William Gerhard undertook a similar research program at Philadelphia, where he obtained an appointment as resident physician at the
Pennsylvania Hospital. The post was awarded to a young physician who
was willing to provide care for the hospital patients between visits of the
regular staff. The resident physician was also allowed to conduct postmortem researches on fatal hospital cases unless there were objections
from the family of the deceased. Using his privileged position, Gerhard
was able to determine that the common continued fever seen at
Philadelphia was identical to Louis's typhoid affection and, further, that
it differed from the remittent or autumnal fever of the United States.[79]

In 1835 Gerhard was appointed a visiting physician at the Philadelphia Hospital and in the winter of 1836 an epidemic of fever broke out in
that city that Gerhard came to believe was the true typhus described by
British medical writers. With the assistance of Pennock, he was able to
distinguish clearly on both symptomatic and pathological evidence the
1836 epidemic of typhus from the common fever or typhoid fever they
had seen before. Gerhard noted several important differences between
typhus and typhoid fever, most obviously that typhus was extremely
contagious; many of the staff of the Philadelphia Hospital contracted the
disease while caring for the sick. The typhus patients had a generalized
rash of red or purple petechiae similar to the rash of measles and quite
distinct from the rose-colored lenticular spots of typhoid. But it was the
absence of the lesions of the Peyer's patches, as well as the constant lack
of secondary postmortem appearance of inflamed mesentery and
enlarged spleen, that convinced Gerhard that typhus was a disease
entirely distinct from typhoid fever.[80]

While Gerhard was working out the distinction between typhoid and
typhus fevers at Philadelphia on the basis of Louis's numerical method,

at the Glasgow Royal Infirmary in Scotland Robert Perry was attempting to discriminate fevers in a less precise, but clinically more acceptable way. At a meeting of the Glasgow Medical Society, Dr. Perry advanced the idea that there were two distinct diseases, typhus fever and dothienenteritis. Typhus fever had been particularly prevalent in Glasgow in 1831, a second hospital having been opened to accommodate the fever patients. In 1835 it was again common. Typhus was believed to be "an idiopathic disease solely produced by contagion . . . only generated in the human body during the course of this idiopathic fever." The clinical course of typhus was generally uniform, and "on the first day from the first attack of headache, rigors, or nausea, a reddish, slightly elevated, but irregular papular or measly eruption is sometimes sparingly, at other times thickly scattered over the trunk and limbs, but rarely appearing on the face." The usual course of typhus "continued for fourteen days from the first attack."

Typhus could be, and often was, complicated by the simultaneous occurrence in the patient of other diseased conditions. Especially common were local inflammations "as of the lungs, the mucous membrane of the stomach and intestines, more particularly the aggregated glands of the ileum, or the membranes of the brain."[81] The local inflammation "kept up" the "febrile action of the system," frequently for another week beyond the original fourteen days.

Dr. Perry believed "that dothienenteritis, or enlargement of the mucous follicles of the smaller intestines, and enlargement and ulceration of the aggregated glands of the lower third of the ileum occur in combination with contagious typhus. It also exists as a disease per se. . . . " The disease possessed its own unique symptom complex, beginning "frequently with diarrhoea, . . . pain in the epigastric, in . . . iliac regions, . . . the abdomen is slightly tumid, and has a puffy feel." Dothienenteritis existed with varying intensity and for varying terms and was distinguished from typhus by the absence of the "frontal headache, low delirium, and decided anorexia, so characteristic of typhus." In his first report of 1835, Dr. Perry noted an absence of eruption on the skin in dothienenteritis, but in 1838 he acknowledged that another eruption sometimes occurred in patients with dothienenteritis "nearly resembling the typhus eruption and which may readily be mistaken for it."[82]

The Glasgow Medical Society appointed a committee to visit Dr. Perry's wards and report on his observations, because his theories "were not considered to be in accordance with the experience of the generality of Members of the Society." The committee deliberated for a year, agreed with Perry on most counts, but reserved final judgment for further study. The society expanded the committee, which after five more months declined to report and suggested that a statistical compilation of fever experience in Glasgow be prepared. This report was drawn up by Robert Cowen. One member of the expanded committee was the surgeon Mr. Charles Ritchie, who would later contribute to the distinction between typhoid and typhus fevers, coining the name enteric fever for the former.[83] Ritchie later recalled that it was Dr. John Home Peebles who provided the suggestion in 1835 that the two eruptions were distinct and that "Dr. Perry . . . followed in 1836. . . ."[84]

In the spring of 1836 Henri C. Lombard of Geneva visited Glasgow on a trip through the British Isles and was surprised by his inability to distinguish the contagious typhus of Glasgow from the "typhus" of Geneva, in which for six years he had observed the lesions of the Peyer's patches at postmortem. He confidently expressed the opinion to his hosts at the Glasgow Royal Infirmary that he could demonstrate upon dissection of a cadaver that "no doubt could exist as to the presence of follicular disease."[85] Yet when the autopsy was performed, no lesions were found. Although shaken, Dr. Lombard believed firmly in the presence of lesions of the Peyer's patches in typhus and at Dublin performed another postmortem examination, a similar failure to find lesions in the small intestine. On leaving Dublin in June 1836, Dr. Lombard wrote to his host, Dr. Robert Graves, describing his sense of confusion, but back in Geneva a month later he wrote a second letter in which he advanced, as a solution to the mystery, the suggestion that there were two similar diseases — Irish typhus, which did not have intestinal lesions, and continental typhus, which did.[86] In the light of Lombard's clinically confusing experience, the reaction of physicians at both Glasgow[87] and Dublin[88] to William Gerhard's 1837 paper on the distinction between Louis's typhoid and British typhus was skeptical. Even so, in the fall of 1837 Gerhard's paper, without cases, was republished in the *Dublin Journal of Medical Science* and an abstract of it appeared in the popular London *Medico-chirurgical Review,* just as William Budd was returning from a third trip to Paris.[89]

There is no information on Budd's studies in 1834–35, but in 1835–36 he spent six months attending the medical practice at the Middlesex Hospital, London, under Francis Hawkins, Thomas Watson, and John Wilson.[90] In the autumn of 1836 he returned a third time to Paris, again studying practical dissection, this time with Dumesnil, as well as surgical pathology with Jean Marjolin and midwifery with C.

Lachapelle. In the winter of 1837 Budd returned to practice with his father at North Tawton, where he reported to his brother that he was "suffering much for want of a stethoscope."[91] There is no evidence that Gerhard's paper on the distinction between typhus and typhoid fevers was available at Paris until September 1838, although he may have sent copies of his articles to Pierre Louis earlier. In the autumn of 1838 Alfred Stillé, who had served as resident physician at the Philadelphia Hospital during the typhus epidemic of 1836–37, went to Paris to complete his medical training. Like Gerhard, Stillé studied with Louis and became a student member of the *Société d'Observation Médicale,* where in the fall of 1838 he presented a paper in which he compared typhoid with typhus fever and showed clearly the differences, clinical and pathological, between the two. Stillé compared the clinical courses of the two diseases and noted the absence of any particular anatomical lesions in post-mortem cases of typhus.[92] As a result of the interest stimulated by Stillé's report, Gerhard's original paper was translated into French and published at Paris.[93]

During 1837–38 William Budd attended the University of Edinburgh medical school but was not impressed. He wrote to his brother Richard, "There is a great parade made of the facilities afforded to the hospital students, but before I had been there three days I was told I *must not ask the Patients any questions* as it interfered with the functions of the clinical clerks; . . . . Of the men I have seen at the Infirmary Dr. Graham is the only one I have a good opinion of: he is far inferior to many I have seen abroad, especially in his mode of investigation."[94]

The work of Louis, of his students, and of independent observers such as H. C. Lombard and Robert Perry drew increasing attention to the differences between fever experience in Britain and seemingly the rest of the western world.

During his period in Edinburgh under William Alison, William Budd began to understand that there were different forms of fever, since he found "the Infirmary here is full of typhus fever." In the spring of 1838 William went to London to stay with his brother George, physician to the *Dreadnought* seamen's hospital, Greenwich, while studying for his medical examinations for the M.D. degree to begin in the summer. The fevers at the *Dreadnought* during this period were "of a lower type than those . . . in Devonshire, . . . in many cases . . . it proves fatal without any local disease. . . ." That summer William visited the hospitals of Dublin, where he found that William Stokes, like Professor Alison at Edinburgh, used wine therapy. He recommended it to George

Budd for the seamen's hospital in the low type of fever as opposed to the fever where the "patches are affected."[95]

Late in 1838 or early in 1839, William returned to North Tawton, where he assisted his father in practice and read. In 1839 Dr. William Henderson, Alison's assistant in Edinburgh and one of Budd's instructors, published an account of the epidemic to which were appended forty-seven autopsy reports by John Reid. The influence of current research on the paper is easy to see. Dr. Henderson encountered a wide variety of clinical symptoms but focused on four varieties of eruption that he thought might be helpful — a common elliptical eruption "not raised in general about the surrounding surface," "punctuations, as if produced by the point of a pen dipped in blood," "large and intensely florid patches," and a papular eruption that rarely existed alone but was seen in combination with the other forms. "Of fifty-three cases in which the figure of the eruptions is specially detailed, thirty-two pertained to the first form; nine of these were closely spotted, seven moderately, sixteen loosely; ten were punctuated, six profusely, four moderately; one presented large patches; five were papular; and five were mixed."[96] However, the statistics of the eruption were not sufficiently precise for Dr. Henderson to delineate clearly a pathology related to other exanthemata or to establish clinically valid differentiations of the fever.

Mr. Reid examined the brain in 43 of the 47 fatal cases autopsied, and "increased effusion of serum within the cranium was observed in 25, or in more than half." In the records from the clinics of these twenty-five cases Reid found symptoms referable to cerebral complications, but similar symptoms had also occurred in some of the remaining eighteen cases, so that he could draw no clear conclusion. Similarly in the study of the lungs he concluded, "It is perfectly obvious that these lesions of the lungs are not the cause of fever, and are not even essential to it; yet they frequently occur during its progress, complicate the disease, and render it more dangerous."[97]

In forty-one of forty-seven cases, John Reid examined the abdominal organs.

> In these 41 cases the elliptical patches of Peyer were apparent and distinctly defined in 24 and in 4 of these the solitary glands of lower part of ileum were also distinctly visible. In 6 cases out of the 41, they were indistinctly defined and scarcely visible; and in 11 cases they could not be distinctly recognized with the naked eye. . . . In 2 only were these elliptical patches very distinctly elevated, and presented any appearance of ulceration. The appearance of the

elliptical patches, which we have described as most commonly observed, . . . is not peculiar to fever, but is not unfrequently observed in various other diseases, ...

The rarity of intestinal lesions in the Edinburgh fever was confirmed by an investigation of the "Register of Dissection" where it was determined that between 1833 and 1837 for 101 cases of fever examined "the elliptical patches are described as being well defined or enlarged in 29. In 7 of the 29 a greater or less degree of ulceration of the patches was observed. . . ."[98]

Reid was surprised to learn from his friend John Goodsir, who was in practice in the village of Anstruther, about thirty miles from Edinburgh, that "the form of fever, as far at least as the post-mortem appearances are concerned, described by Louis and Chomel," was quite common. The village averaged about one hundred cases of fever annually. In 1838–39 sixteen had died, and Goodsir had obtained permission to autopsy ten; all had lesions of the Peyer's patches. John Reid offered no explanation of the fever accompanied by lesions of Peyer's patches at Anstruther but presented it as "an interesting and instructive fact."[99]

In 1838 Alexander Tweedie and Robert Christison, who had been a classmate of Tweedie at the Edinburgh medical school and who in 1838 was a medical teacher at Edinburgh, visited Paris to tour the hospitals. At the Hôtel Dieu, where Pierre Louis now gave clinical lectures, Tweedie and Christison discussed fever with the French pathologist. Louis reportedly admitted his belief in two diseases — typhoid fever and British typhus — a belief he accepted in print in the second edition of his work on typhoid fever in 1841. He admitted to Tweedie and Christison that he had no personal experience with British typhus but had assumed in the 1820s that he was dealing with the same disease in Paris that the British had described.[100]

Tweedie and Christison, having experienced the clinical realities of practice in London and Edinburgh, could not accept that there were two distinct diseases, one characterized by intestinal lesions and the other without them. They extended an invitation to Louis to visit them or to send a student to their hospitals to examine their cases. After Stillé's report and after he had read Gerhard's paper, Louis took advantage of Tweedie's offer. Early in 1839 an American physician, George Cheyne Shattuck, having completed three years of postgraduate training with Louis, was ready to return home to Boston. Shattuck had graduated M.D. from Harvard in 1835, having studied medicine under James

Jackson, Sr. He had observed typhoid fever at Boston and at Paris and
had become adept at diagnosis. Shattuck went to London and for two
months, February and March 1839, studied fever at the London Fever
Hospital. After he returned home, he published his thirteen cases from
London. He had performed careful postmortems on each fatal case after
the manner of Louis and had divided the patients into two classes — three
cases of fever accompanied by abdominal symptoms, rose colored spots,
and diarrhea in which at autopsy Shattuck had found the characteristic
lesions of the Peyer's patches, and ten cases in which there were no
obvious abdominal symptoms and in which he had found at autopsy no
evidence of disease in the small bowel.[101]

Nevertheless, Shattuck's retrospective report, in which he confirmed
or corrected diagnosis by the results of postmortem analysis, may be
misleading. Tweedie recalled in 1860, "Soon after my visit to Paris, Dr.
Shattuck . . . came to London, if not with the express object of investigating the pathology of fevers, this subject, at all events, engaged a good
deal of his attention. At the request of Louis, he visited the wards of the
Fever Hospital, in which he spent much time, and therefore had the
opportunity of observing the cases as they were admitted; and I well
remember the difficulty he felt in diagnosing the two forms presented to
his observation."[102]

After completing his M.D. degree in 1838, William Budd repeatedly
spent time in London, where through his older brother George Budd he
gained entry to the medical world of that city and was able to expand his
medical knowledge further. Almost certainly he would have visited the
Fever Hospital, and he may have met George Shattuck; he learned of
James Jackson's recent publication of typhoid fever cases from the
Massachusetts General Hospital, although he did not see a copy. By the
summer of 1839 he had returned to North Tawton, where he practiced
with his father or in his father's place for two years. During his time in
Devonshire, he experienced the epidemic of typhoid fever that was so
instrumental in shaping his ideas of the contagiousness of that disease,
and he competed for the Thackeray Prize of the Provincial Medical and
Surgical Association.[103] In July 1839 an epidemic of fever broke out at
North Tawton that convinced Budd of the contagious and specific nature
of the disease called by Louis typhoid fever. He was writing his essay as
early as August but needed some notes and books from London. By
early December he was "a good way on with my essay" but "for want of
time many of the topics will not receive the development which might be
given. . . ." Budd described his essay:

I begin by discussing the question touching the identity of the two
forms of fever. I leave that question undecided but with a strong
presumption that the forms are *specifically* different. . . . On the
strength of that presumption I consider it necessary to make a
separate inquiry into the causes of the two forms of fever & I divide
the subject accordingly. I treat first the form with ulcerations,
introduce a succinct narrative of the N. Tawton epidemic and make
a lengthened commentary. I prove the contagious nature of the
disease most abundantly & then discuss the facts and arguments for
& against spontaneous origin — I show that in our present state of
knowledge we are not qualified to decide that point, much less
therefore to determine by what process other than contagion the
fever agent may be generated. I hold up the absurdity of attributing
the production of an agent so specific in nature to such a variety of
circumstances as are currently named in books. . . . I add that we
have the same grounds for assigning the poisons of sm. pox,
measles, and scarlatine to a similar number of circumstances. . . . I
illustrate by apt quotations from Bateman, Willan, & Parent
Duchatelet the inadequacy of the production of fever of the circumstances that have most repute in that line. Considering this form of
fever therefore as a disease propagated by contagion I next take a
lengthened and analytical review of the circumstances that may
affect its spread, treating of these circumstances as they may affect
the poison, the person exposed, or both. . . . In the next and last
chapter I shall treat of the form without ulcerations, not so much at
length because many of the considerations in the former chapter
apply to contagious diseases in general. . . .[104]

William Budd finished his essay and submitted it, but he did not win
the Thackeray Prize in 1840. His idea that there were two distinct
diseases as well as his belief in the essentially contagious nature of fever
were too revolutionary and, it must be admitted, inadequately supported. The winner of the Thackeray Prize was William Davidson, a
physician of the Glasgow Royal Infirmary, whose essay was published
by John Forbes, one of the adjudicating committee, in the *British and
Foreign Medical Review*.

Dr. Davidson defined three varieties of continued fever — typhus,
fibricula or simple fever, and gastric or intestinal fever — which seemed
"to be distinct species of disease, differing in their symptoms, causes, and
laws. . . ." Of the other varieties of continued fever mentioned in the
literature Davidson wrote, "Many of these have been found, on investigation, only particular varieties, in place of being distinct species. This
has been particularly the case with typhus, the most prevalent kind of
continued fever in this country. . . . The pathology of typhus, however,

of late years has been considerably advanced; and it is now established, that this disease may be either simple or complicated, with organic affections of one or all of the different cavities of the body."[105]

Typhus for Davidson was the disease so named by "our standard authors upon this subject," but he did wish to draw attention to the fact that the disease had "a distinctive characteristic, viz., the eruption, which is present in none of the others, and which is now almost universally acknowledged as decisive of its existence." He used the British meaning of the word *typhoid* — i.e., typhuslike, throughout the essay. In explaining the eruption on the skin, for example, he wrote, "The large majority of patients who have decidedly the general typhoid symptoms, are more or less spotted with this efflorescence."[106] He accepted that typhus could exist in a simple form or with complications of various organ systems, but such complications were secondary and did not enter into the study of causes.

Davidson acknowledged the diversity of opinion that existed on the cause of continued fevers but affirmed that the majority believed it to be "propagated by contagion." He used the analogy of the exanthemata to establish that typhus fever was also contagious, "propagated only by the *effluvia* which are generated by the patient." He avoided all speculation on the origin or ultimate origin of typhus contagion and devoted his attention to establishing its contagiousness based on the experience reported by authors and his own experience in Glasgow. Davidson leaned heavily on the reports of the 1816–1819 epidemics, particularly those in Ireland as collected by Barker and Cheyne. He cited other standard British authorities, including Alexander Tweedie and William Alison, and French writings on the typhoid fever of Louis. He credited Pierre Bretonneau with transforming French opinion on the contagiousness of typhus: "The majority of French physicians are of opinion that typhoid fever is not contagious, and their belief was almost universal until M. Bretonneau published a contrary opinion." The evidences used by Davidson are the standard arguments from the exanthemata experience: "1. The contagion can be traced in families, hospitals, schools, &c., . . . 2. They only affect persons once during their lives. 3. They are characterized by an eruption. . . ."[107] In support of the second point, that contagious diseases affect persons only once, he cited the evidence of H. C. Lombard and Robert Perry, both of whom had made unsuccessful efforts to establish that typhus was distinct from typhoid fever. On the prevalence of the rash Davidson cited Louis and Chomel.

Gastric or intestinal fever was, like simple fever, "a febrile affection . . . of an ephemeral kind. . . ." Davidson suspected it was the result of "the existence of solid excrementitious matter in the cells of the ileum. . . . It may be distinguished from typhus at the commencement by ascertaining the antecedent circumstances of the patient, and by the state of his bowels and abdomen." But Davidson acknowledged that such means were not always sufficient; if the attack were of typically short duration, as it was "in the great majority of cases," the problem was solved. There remained the problem inherited in some measure from Perry and Lombard, which Davidson expressed as follows:

> In some instances, however, particularly when diarrhoea is present, the attack is prolonged for a week or two, and sometimes for two or three weeks. In some of these cases there is a tendency to peritonitis, while in others there is reason to suspect some enlargement or ulceration of the glands of the intestines. We are quite aware that such cases, which are not of frequent occurrence, might be called typhus fever without eruption; and in the present state of our diagnostic means this question cannot be solved in a satisfactory manner. . . .[108]

Davidson challenged the various alleged sources of continued fevers in putrid effluvia, exhalations from humans in dirty or crowded conditions, in filth of impure air, or in malaria. All such circumstances could and did favor the diffusion of continued fevers and contributed to the communication of fever from the sick to the healthy but could not in themselves cause the fever.

Finally, Davidson discussed briefly the question of the identity of typhus and typhoid fever. He argued that those French authorities who believed typhoid to be a different disease, particularly Chomel and Louis, had failed to take into proper account the similarities. Davidson stressed the similarities between the symptoms described for typhoid fever by the French and those acknowledged to be part of the clinical picture of typhus in Britain. He quoted H. C. Lombard's clinical difficulties in Glasgow and Dublin and even Chomel's reference to having observed patients in 1814–15 in whom all the symptoms of typhoid were observed but who did not exhibit the typhoid lesion at postmortem. Davidson similarly quotes from H. C. Lombard and William Gerhard to show that there are numerous pathological similarities between the cases described as two diseases by those pathologists, completely missing the point that it was the constant differences that were considered important by the new school of anatomic pathology.

The clinical realities are the most telling point, however. "It is quite evident that Drs. Lombard and Gerhard lay almost the whole weight of the diagnosis of typhus from the typhoid fever, upon the lesions of the intestinal follicles observed in the latter disease, for the almost identity of their symptoms during life are admitted; and is there any British practitioner that could distinguish those cases of eruptive typhus that had diseased follicles from those that had not? [109]

The terms of Davidson's 1839 question clearly suggested that he thought no responsible practitioner would differentiate typhoid from typhus fever; and in 1839 very few practitioners were able or willing to make the distinction. During the 1840s, however, the number grew steadily, in part as a result of continued research, but most importantly in response to disease experience. Clear-cut epidemic experiences help differentiate among continued fevers, and, despite confusion, practitioners began to realize the pathological, etiological, and epidemiological implications of such experiences. Among the earliest to appreciate the importance of the concept of specificity in the study of fevers and to understand its impact on etiology and public health was William Budd. His Thackeray Prize essay illustrates both his appreciation and his confusion and as such has great interest for historians of medicine and is of importance in the development of a clearer understanding of the research on fevers in Victorian Britain.

NOTES

1. Lloyd Stevenson, "Examplary Diseases: The Typhoid Pattern," *J. Hist. Med.,* 1982, *37,* 159–81.

2. The process of differentiation among fevers had progressed considerably prior to the early Victorian period; periodic, particularly intermittent, fevers had been separated out of the generalized class fever by all but a few practitioners. The exanthemata had been distinguished early in the nineteenth century — see Thomas Bateman, *Delineations of Cutaneous Diseases: Exhibiting the Characteristic Appearances of the Principal Genera and Species Comprised in the Classification of the Late Dr. Willan* (London: Longman, Hurst, Rees, Orme and Brown, 1817) or idem, *A Practical Synopsis of Cutaneous Diseases, According to the Arrangement of Dr. Willan* (London: Longman, Hurst, Rees, Orme and Brown, 1813).

There were a variety of names for many diseases in the nineteenth century. The disease known in America and France as typhoid fever was called abdominal typhus in Germany and enteric fever in Great Britain. William Budd suggested the name intestinal fever.

3. Charles Creighton, *A History of Epidemics in Britain,* 2 vols. (Cambridge: Cambridge University Press, 1891–1894), 2: 211.

4. Royston Lambert, *Sir John Simon, 1816–1904, and English Social Administration* (London: MacGibbon & Kee, 1963), pp. 618–19.

5. Arthur Newsholme, *The Story of Modern Preventive Medicine* (London: Ballière, Tindall and Cox, 1929), pp. 88–105.

6. Robert Koch, "Die Bekämpfung des Typhus," *Veröff. Geb. Milit. Sanit. Wes.*, 1903, *21*, 1–21. Charles A. Cameron, "Report on the Typhoid Fever Epidemic in Dublin," *Brit. Med. J.*, 1891, *2*, 1167–68, expressed concern over the frequency of typhoid fever in Dublin but could not explain it. Charles A. Cameron, "Extracts from the Cavendish Lecture on Some Points in the Etiology of Typhoid Fever," *Brit. Med. J.*, 1892, *1*, 1244–45, mentioned the belief that oysters caused typhoid fever but did not believe the spread by oysters a sufficient explanation and looked to the soil and Rodet and Roux's virulent activation theory of the typhoid bacillus as an altered strain of Escherich's colon bacillus. H. W. Conn, "The Oyster Epidemic of Typhoid Fever at Wesleyan University," *Med. Rec.*, 1894, *46*, 743–46, clearly recognizes shellfish as an agent, demonstrating the presence of the bacteria for the first time.

Wesley W. Spink, *Infectious Diseases; Prevention and Treatment in the Nineteenth and Twentieth Centuries* (Minneapolis: University of Minnesota Press, 1978), pp. 242–43.

7. William Budd, *Typhoid Fever: Its Nature, Mode of Spreading, and Prevention* (1873, reprinted New York: American Public Health Association, 1931).

8. William Budd, "Intestinal Fever Essentially Contagious," *Lancet*, 1859, *2*, 4–5, 28–30, 55–56, 80–82, 131–33, 207–10, 432–33, 458–59; 1860, *1*, 187–90, 239–40; the note is on page 5.

9. E. W. Goodall, *William Budd, M.D. Edin., F.R.S., the Bristol Physician and Epidemiologist* (Bristol: Arrowsmith, 1936), pp. 40–54. Margaret Pelling, *Cholera, Fever, and English Medicine, 1825–1865* (Oxford: Oxford University Press, 1978), pp. 281–82, particularly n. 3.

10. Dale C. Smith, "William Budd Manuscript at the National Library of Medicine," *J. Hist. Med.*, 1980, *35*, 318–19; see also the Appendix.

11. Ernest Little, comp., *History of the British Medical Association, 1832–1932* (London: BMA, 1932), pp. 313–14, and W. H. McMenemey, *The Life and Times of Sir Charles Hastings, Founder of the British Medical Association* (Edinburgh: Livingstone, 1959), pp. 100, 182, 206, 324.

12. "Proceedings at the First Anniversary Meeting of the Provincial Medical and Surgical Association, at the Bristol Infirmary," *Trans. Prov. Med. Surg. Assoc.*, 1834, *2*, xxiii–xxix.

13. Ibid., p. xxix.

14. "Report of the Council, 1834," *Trans. Prov. Med. Surg. Assoc.*, 1835, *3*, 6–9.

15. "Proceedings at the Fifth Anniversary Meeting of the Provincial Medical and Surgical Association, Held at Cheltenham," *Trans. Prov. Med. Surg. Assoc.*, 1837, *6*(1), 1–46.

16. Ibid., p. 19.

17. Ibid., pp. 25, 33–34.

18. "Thackeray Prize," *Trans. Prov. Med. Surg. Assoc.*, 1838, *6*(2), unnumbered page appended to the volume.

19. "Proceedings at the Sixth Anniversary Meeting of the Provincial Medical and Surgical Association, Held at Bath," *Trans. Prov. Med. Surg. Assoc.*, 1839, *7*, 5–70.

20. "Proceedings at the Eighth Anniversary Meeting of the Provincial Medical and Surgical Association, Held at Southampton," *Trans. Prov. Med. Surg. Assoc.*, 1841, *9*, 5–56. I have assumed that Dr. Conolly remained Dr. John Conolly, coeditor with Dr. John Forbes of the *British and Foreign Medical Review* and member of the prize subject-selection committee; McMenemey, *Sir Charles Hastings*, p. 206, identifies him as William

Conolly, an elder brother and also a member of the association. Both were Edinburgh M.D.s (William, 1818; John, 1821) who had spent time in France.

21. "Proceedings," (n.20), p. 25.

22. William Davidson, "Essay on the Sources and Mode of Propagation of the Continued Fevers of Great Britain and Ireland," *Brit. For. Med. Rev.,* 1841, *11,* appendix pp. 1–80.

23. George Eliot, *Middlemarch* and *George Eliot's Middlemarch Notebooks: A Transcription,* John Clark Pratt and Victor A. Neufeldt, eds. (Berkeley: University of California Press, 1979).

24. Pelling, *Cholera, Fever and English Medicine.*

25. Biographical information on William Budd is available in several sources but the best is Goodall, *William Budd.* More recently Pelling, *Cholera, Fever and English Medicine* has examined Budd's scientific work in some detail. Where other sources are not cited, I have followed Goodall.

26. W. F. Bynum, "Cullen and the Study of Fevers in Britain, 1760–1820," in W. F. Bynum and V. Nutton, eds., *Theories of Fever from Antiquity to the Enlightenment* (London: Wellcome Institute, 1981), pp. 135–47; W. F. Bynum, "Hospital, Disease, and Community: the London Fever Hospital, 1801–1850," in Charles Rosenberg, ed., *Healing and History* (New York: Science History Publications, 1979), pp. 97–115; Ulrich Tröller, "Quantification in British Medicine and Surgery, 1750–1830, with Special Reference to Its Introduction into Therapeutics," Ph.D. thesis, University of London, 1978.

27. Thomas Bateman, *A Succinct Account of the Contagious Fevers of This Country* (London: Longman, Hurst, Rees, Orme and Brown, 1818); Edward Percival, *Practical Observations on the Treatment, Pathology, and Prevention of Typhous Fever* (Bath: Cruttwell, 1819).

28. Percival, *Practical Observations,* pp. 49–51.

29. Ibid., p. 62.

30. Bateman, *A Succinct Account,* pp. 22, 30, 33.

31. "The Epidemic Fever," *Edin. Med. Surg. J.,* 1821, *17,* 620–34.

32. Henry Clutterbuck, *Observations on the Prevention and Treatment of the Epidemic Fever at Present Prevailing in the Metropolis, etc.* (London: Longman, Hurst, Rees, Orme and Brown, 1819).

33. Owsei Temkin, "The Role of Surgery in the Rise of Modern Medical Thought," in idem, *The Double Face of Janus* (Baltimore: The Johns Hopkins University Press, 1977), pp. 487–96.

34. Henry Clutterbuck, *An Essay on Pyrexia* (London: S. Highley, 1837), p. iii.

35. *Dictonary of National Biography* s.v. "Clutterbuck, Henry."

36. Clutterbuck, *Pyrexia,* pp. iii–v. On the bloodletting revolution see Peter H. Niebyl, "The English Bloodletting Revolution, or Modern Medicine before 1850," *Bull. Hist. Med.,* 1977, *51,* 464–83.

37. Clutterbuck, *Pyrexia,* p. iii.

38. Bateman, *A Succinct Account,* p. x.

39. Admission tickets from the lectures for which Budd registered in Paris are preserved in the Budd Papers, London School of Tropical Medicine.

40. François Joseph Victor Broussais, *Histoire des phlegmasies ou inflammations chronique* (Paris: Gabon, 1808).

41. Esmond Long, "The First Text of Pathology Published in America," *Arch. Path.,* 1930, *9,* 898–909.

42. Frank Mann and Ruth Mann, "Laennec as a Critical Pathologist," *J. Hist. Med.*, 1981, *36*, 446-54.

43. William Boyd, *A Textbook of Pathology* (Philadelphia: Lea & Febiger, 1970), p. 800.

44. R. T. H. Laennec, *Traité de l'auscultation médiate*, 2 vols. (Paris: Brosson, 1826), 1: 280.

45. M. A. Petit and E. R. A. Serres, *Traité de la fièvre entéromésentérique* (Paris: Hacquart, 1813).

46. A. Chomel, *Des fièvre et des maladies pestilentielles* (Paris: Crochard, 1821).

47. C. Hewett, "Cases Showing the Frequency of the Occurrence of Follicular Ulceration on the Mucous Membrane of the Intestines, During the Progress of Idiopathic Fever, . . ." *London Med. Phys. J.*, 1826, *56*, 97-114, 241-51.

48. Richard Bright, *Reports of Medical Cases*, 2 vols. (London: Longman, 1827-31), 1: 178, 183.

49. Pierre Bretonneau, *Traité de la dothinentérie et de la spécificité* (Paris: Vigot Frères, 1922).

50. Armand Trousseau, "Pierre Bretonneau," *Union Médicale*, 1862, *13*, 237.

51. Armand Trousseau, "De la maladie à laquelle M. Bretonneau, médecin de l'hôpital de Tours, a donné le nom de dothinentérie, ou de dothinentérite," *Arch. Gén. Méd.*, 1826, *10*, 67-78, 169-216.

52. Trousseau cited the work of Andral, Rayer, Billard, Hutin, Breschet and Chauffard d'Avignon, ibid., pp. 67, 204.

53. Laennec's M.D. thesis in 1804 was on Hippocratic ideas of fever and their usefulness in his time, while in 1839 Emile Littré translated the Hippocratic corpus into French for its medical usefulness. Chomel's *Fièvre* cited with equal authority observations from the eighteenth and nineteenth centuries.

54. Pierre Louis, *Recherches anatomique-pathologique sur la phthisie* (Paris: Gabon, 1825).

55. Pierre Louis, "Du croup considéré chez l'adulte," *Arch. Gén. Méd.*, 1824, *4*, 5-30, 369-86.

56. Pierre Louis, "Observations relatives aux perforations spontanées de l'intestin grêle dans les maladies aiguës," *Arch. Gén. Méd.*, 1823, *1*, 17-49.

57. Pierre Louis, *Recherches anatomiques, pathologiques et thérapeutiques sur la maladie connue sous le nom de gastro-entérite, fièvre putride, etc.*, 2 vols. (Paris: Baillière, 1829).

58. E. W. Goodall, *William Budd.*

59. John Armstrong, *Practical Illustrations of Typhus Fever, etc.*, 3rd ed. (Philadelphia: Webster, 1822); see also Thomas Bateman, *A Succinct Account* for a similar view.

60. William T. Gairdner, "Dr. Alison," in idem, *The Physician as Naturalist* (Glasgow: Maclehose, 1889), pp. 388-430.

61. Leonard G. Wilson, "Fevers and Science in Early Nineteenth Century Medicine," *J. Hist. Med.*, 1978, *33*, 386-407.

62. "Report of Diseases Treated at the Edinburgh New Town Dispensary, from June 1st to September 1st, and from September 1st to December 1st, 1816," *Edin. Med. Surg. J.*, 1817, *13*, 117-24; "Report of Diseases Treated at the Edinburgh New Town Dispensary, from December 1st, 1816 to March 1st, 1817," *Edin. Med. Surg. J.*, 1817, *13*, 245-49; "Report of Diseases Treated at the Edinburgh New Town Dispensary, from March 1st to June 1st, 1817," *Edin. Med. Surg. J.*, 1817, *13*, 398-404; "Report of Diseases Treated at the Edinburgh New Town Dispensary, from June 1st to September 1st, 1817," *Edin. Med. Surg. J.*, 1817, *13*, 521-27; "Report of Diseases Treated at the Edinburgh New

Town Dispensary, from September 1st to December 1st, 1817," *Edin. Med. Surg. J.*, 1817, *14*, 120–26.

63. William Pulteney Alison, "Observations on the Epidemic Fever Now Prevalent among the Lower Orders in Edinburgh," *Edin. Med. Surg. J.*, 1827, *28*, 233–63.

64. Ibid., p. 245.

65. Ibid., p. 257.

66. Ibid., pp. 258–59.

67. Alexander Tweedie, *Clinical Illustrations of Fever* (London: Whittaker, 1830), p. 10.

68. Ibid., pp. 22–26, 33.

69. Ibid., p. 23.

70. Ibid., p. 39.

71. Ibid., p. 40.

72. Auguste Chomel, *Leçons de clinique médicale*, 2 vols. (Paris: Baillière, 1834). All of volume one is devoted to typhoid fever.

73. Gabriel Andral, *Clinique médicale*, 5 vols. (Paris: Cavellin, 1829–33).

74. François Broussais, *Examen des doctrines médicales et les systèmes de nosologie*, 3d ed., 4 vols. (Paris: Méquignon-Marvis, 1829–33); P. Louis, *Examen de l'Examen de M. Broussais* (Paris: Ballière, 1834).

75. William Budd to his brother Samuel Budd, 6 December 1833, p.m., Budd Letters, Wellcome Institute, London.

76. Russell M. Jones, ed., *The Parisian Education of an American Surgeon: Letters of Jonathan Mason Warren (1832–1835)* (Philadelphia: American Philosophical Society, 1978).

77. Wilson, "Fevers and science."

78. Dale C. Smith, "Gerhard's Distinction between Typhoid and Typhus, and its Reception in America 1833–1860," *Bull. Hist. Med.*, 1980, *54*, 368–85.

79. Ibid.; William Wood Gerhard, "Report of Cases Treated in the Medical Wards of the Pennsylvania Hospital," *Am. J. Med. Sci.*, 1835, *15*, 321–41; *16*, 35–37.

80. William W. Gerhard, "On the Typhus Fever Which Occurred in Philadelphia in the Spring and Summer of 1836," *Am. J. Med. Sci.*, 1836, *19*, 289–322; 1837, *20*, 289–322.

81. Archibald L. Goodall, "Glasgow's Place in the Distinction between Typhoid and Typhus Fevers," *Bull. Hist. Med.*, 1954, *28*, 140–53. Also Robert Perry, "On Contagion, Particularly the Typhus Contagion," *Medical Essays of the Glasgow Medical Society*, vol. 22, session 8, 7 April 1835; "Report of Commission to Visit Wards of the Fever Hospital under the Charge of Dr. Perry," *Medical Essays of the Glasgow Medical Society*, vol. 23, session 11, 17 May 1836 in the Library, Royal College of Physicians and Surgeons of Glasgow.

82. Robert Perry, "Statistics of Typhus Fever," *Medical Essays of the Glasgow Medical Society*, vol. 25, session 8, 20 March 1838 in the Library, Royal College of Physicians and Surgeons of Glasgow.

83. Archibald Goodall, "Glasgow's Place," pp. 143, 151.

84. Charles Ritchie, "Clinical Lecture on Typhus and Continued Fever," *Glasgow Med. J.*, 1855, *3*, 16–36.

85. H. C. Lombard, "Observations Suggested by a Comparison of the Post Mortem Appearances Produced by Typhous Fever in Dublin, Paris, and Geneva," *Dublin J. Med. Sci.*, 1836, *10*, 17–24.

86. H. C. Lombard, "Second Letter from Doctor Lombard to Doctor Graves on the Subject of Typhous Fever," *Dublin J. Med. Sci.*, 1836, *10*, 101–5.

87. *Medical Essays of the Glasgow Medical Society* in which five physicians read papers on fevers between 1838 and 1841, most in opposition to the ideas of Perry, Lombard, and Gerhard. Dr. Cheyne at meeting of 16 January 1838, Dr. Weir on 5 February 1839, Dr. Maxwell on 15 October 1839, Mr. Lyon on 4 February 1840, Dr. Hannay on 16 March 1841. The doctrine of essential unity of fever seems to have been broken in Glasgow by the 1843 relapsing fever.

88. William Stokes, "A Discourse on the Life and Works of the Late Robert James Graves, M.D., F.R.S.," *Med. Times Gaz.*, 1854, *8*, 1–5.

89. William W. Gerhard, "On the Typhous Fever, Which Occurred at Philadelphia in the Spring and Summer of 1836, . . ." *Dublin J. Med. Sci.*, 1838, *12*, 148–61; "Fever in America and Ireland, 1. Philadelphia Hospital," *Med. Chir. Rev.*, 1837, *27*, 553–57.

90. In a letter to George, 13 December 1837, William asks for the "minutes for the winter of 1834–35 which was that in which we wrote our cases at the Middlesex," suggesting the possibility of a longer period at the Middlesex Hospital. Budd Letters. The surviving certificate is for six months, a year later.

91. William Budd to George Budd, 14 February 1837, Budd Letters.

92. Alfred Stillé, "Table of Comparison between Typhus and Typhoid Fever," *Penn. Univ. Med. Bull.*, 1904–05, *17*, 63–74.

93. Wilson, "Fevers and Science," p. 404.

94. William Budd to Richard Budd, from Edinburgh, n.d., postmarked 27 November 1837, Budd Letters.

95. Ibid.; George and William Budd to Richard Budd, n.d., labeled "1st yr. at Dreadnought," Budd Letters.

96. William Henderson, "Report on the Epidemic Fever of Edinburgh. An Account of the Symptoms and Treatment," *Edin. Med. Surg. J.*, 1839, *52*, 429–48.

97. John Reid, "Analysis and Details of Forty-seven Inspections After Death," *Edin. Med. Surg. J.*, 1839, *52*, 448–62.

98. Ibid., p. 459.

99. Ibid.

100. Alexander Tweedie, "Lectures on Fevers," *Lancet*, 1860, *1*, 53–56.

101. George C. Shattuck, "On the Continued Fevers of Great Britain," *Med. Exam.*, 1840, *3*, 133–40, 149–54.

102. Tweedie, "Lectures on fever," p. 53.

103. Goodall, *William Budd*, pp. 36–37.

104. William Budd to George Budd, 6 December 1839. Budd Letters.

105. Davidson, "Essay on Continued Fevers," p. 1.

106. Ibid., pp. 1–2.

107. Ibid., pp. 1–2, 9.

108. Ibid., p. 36.

109. Ibid., p. 79.

AN ESSAY

ON THE CAUSES
AND MODE OF PROPAGATION
OF THE COMMON
CONTINUED FEVERS OF
GREAT BRITAIN
AND IRELAND.

DECEMBER 1839
[WILLIAM BUDD]

The interesting bearing of symmetrical affections on therapeutics —

Statistics in medicine no great engine of discovery — good for testing theories — the facts numbered not quantitative in their nature

Points for further investigation

1. The relation of the affection of Peyer glands to the Typhus (contagious) fevers of Gt Bn & Id
2. Does the presence of this affection constitute a specific division of fevers?
3. The relations of the Exanthem to Typhus — and its accurate history & description
4. A comparison of the propagation (the <u>laws of</u>) of diseases avowed contagious — S.pox, measles, scarlet f. — with that of typhus
5. The history (or laws) of typhus in relation to the power of an attack to produce insusceptibility to a second — & its relation in this respect to other contagious diseases
6. The limits of the period when the contagion from an individual begins & ceases —
7. The extreme limit of the period during which contagion may remain in <u>fomites</u> — (from facts)

Contagion

This subject is one of the first magnitude that falls to the discussion of a physician. By it the operations of fleets and armies are overthrown on a sudden & the best conceived plans rendered abortive —

Blane [1]

1. [Sir Gilbert Blane; I have been unable to locate this passage as a quotation from Blane's works.]

If it were asked what is the cause of the Jail fever? it would in
general be readily replied "the want of fresh air and cleanliness." But
as I have found in some prisons abroad, cells and dungeons as
offensive as any I have observed in this country, where, however
this distemper is unknown, I am obliged to look out for some
additional cause of its production.

Howard on Lazurettoes.
Page 231 2nd Edition [2]

Felix qui potuit rerum cognoscere causas — Virgil [3]

2. [John Howard, *An Account of the Principal Lazarettos in Europe, etc.*, 2d ed. (London, 1791).]
3. [*Georgics* 2, 490. This quotation was added to the manuscript after its original submission.]

CHAPTER 1ST

Introductory.

Question: — "The investigation of the sources of the common continued fevers of Great Britain and Ireland, and the ascertaining of the circumstances which favour the diffusion of these diseases, and also those circumstances which may have a tendency to render them communicable from one person to another."

In the consideration of this question I shall assume that the words "common continued fevers" were [2] intended to designate those forms of essential fever, commonly called typhoid or typhous fever, and which are always more or less prevalent in Great Britain and Ireland, and furnish in the Metropolis, and in some other large towns a constant supply of sick to fever hospitals.

The great annual mortality from these fevers in the United Kingdom; — the preference they affect for persons[4] in the prime of

---

4. † The heads of families almost uniformly became victims ["]while the rest escaped. . . . The widows and the orphans, who are so numerous in every quarter, can bear [a] sad testimony to the truth of this well known observation.["] Dr. Bracken in Barker & Cheyne, vol:1.p:198.

[John King Bracken, M.D., one of the physicians of the Waterford Fever Hospital. His report, "Medical Report of the Fever Hospital of the City and of the County of Waterford, during the Epidemic Fever of the Years 1817, 1818, and 1819," is in F. Barker and J. Cheyne, *An Account of the Rise, Progress, and Decline of the Fever Lately Epidemical in Ireland,* 2 vols. (Dublin, 1821), 1, 182–280.]

A fever which consigns thousands to the grave consigns tens of thousands to a worse fate, to hopeless poverty, for fever cuts off the parents leaving the wretched offspring to fill the future ranks of prostitution, mendicancy & crime — Harty's Sketch

[William Harty. *An Historical Sketch of the Causes, Progress, Extent and Mortality of the Contagious Fever Epidemic in Ireland, etc.,* 2 vols. (Dublin, 1820). This same quotation is included in William Budd, "On Intestinal Fever: Its Mode of Propagation," *Lancet,* 1856, *2,* 694.]

In the last situation in which I have seen fever prevailing epidemically in Edinburgh I find, on inquiry that 5 families out of the inhabitants of 12 rooms in the 2 upper flats of the house have been rendered fatherless by it. Alison. Management of the Poor in Scotland p. 4

[William P. Alison, *Observations on the Management of the Poor in Scotland and its Effects on the Health of the Great Towns* (Edinburgh, 1840).]

From returns made in 1838 by the Medical officers of 20 unions and parishes in the metropolis, it appeared that 13,972 cases of claims to relief on grounds of destitution were created during that year by attacks of fever alone, and that in 1,281 cases the attacks proved fatal. The general deaths from fever in the metropolis during that year appear from the Summary of the Superintendent of

life; — the frequency of their outbreak in epidemics that spread through large masses of population, and destroy or disable vast numbers of the working class; — are sufficient evidence of their importance in a social point of view, and of the interest that must attach to inquiry into their causes and mode of propagation.

Accordingly we find that this inquiry has been taken up by [3] a great number of eminent physicians and has more than once engaged the especial attention of Parliament.

Still however much discrepancy of opinion prevails, both regarding the causes and mode of propagation of these fevers, as may be seen by reference to the latest and best works on the subject: and it is apparent from the variety and frequent incongruity of the circumstances which writers of acknowledged authority have set down, without order or distinction, as causes of these fevers, that the whole subject is still involved in deep obscurity. This is mainly owing to the abstruse nature of the subject and the peculiar difficulty of obtaining evidence needful for its elucidation. Much confusion has also been introduced by those engaged in the inquiry, from general want of perception to the kind of evidence needed; and still more, from want of discriminating [4] between forms of fever which differ in many material if not essential characters.

It has long been ascertained that a large proportion of those who die of fever in London, Edinburgh and Dublin do not exhibit that special alteration of the intestinal follicles, which on account of its constancy in Fever in Paris is there regarded as the anatomical character of the disease.

The absence of this and of any special lesion of the intestines is sometimes pretty uniformly observed through the whole course of an Epidemic; as in that for Example of which Dr. Alison has given a narrative in the 28th Volume of the Edinburgh Medical and Surgical Journal.[5] In other Epidemics the well [5] known specific alteration of

---

Registrar's returns to have been 5,634. Letter from the poor law commissioners to the Metropolitan Board of Guardians Nov. 11, — 40.

[Great Britain, Poor Law Commissioners, *Seventh Annual Report*, "Appendix A, Number 8, Sanitary Inquiry — Circular Letter to Boards of Guardians, 11 November 1840," pp. 101–3, *PP*, 1841, *11*, 201 ff. also quoted by Budd, "On Intestinal Fever."]

5. (1) See also Med:Gazette vol:19. p. 570. (Clinical Lectures by Dr. Graves) and the Edinburgh Medical & Surgical Journal, Oct. 1839, for a paper on Fever by Drs. Henderson and J. Reid.

[William Pulteney Alison, "Observations on the Epidemic Fever Now Prevalent among the Lower Orders in Edinburgh," *Edin. Med. Surg. J.*, 1827, *28*, 233–63; Robert Graves, "Clinical Lectures Delivered at the Meath Hospital and County of Dublin Infirmary — Maculated Fever and Typhus without Maculae," *London Med. Gaz.*, 1836, *19*, 570–71; William Henderson and John Reid, "Report on the Epidemic Fever of Edinburgh," *Edin. Med. Surg. J.*, 1839, *52*, 429–62.]

Peyer's patches for which the writings of French physicians have acquired such notoriety; is observed as uniformly.

The question therefore naturally arises whether two series of cases which differ in so material a point of their morbid anatomy, be mere varieties of one disease, or on the contrary, examples of two diseases specifically different from one another.

There are many acute diseases other than fever, that vary greatly in type from one epidemic to another, but none exhibit in their different types a difference of anatomical character at all equal in moment to [6] that just referred to. The discussion of the question arising out of this difference is therefore an indispensable preliminary to any inquiry into the [6] causes of fever, and I shall enter upon it without further preface.

The first point which strikes us is that if the two forms of fever above referred to be merely varieties of one disease, it is very remarkable that one of these varieties, — that, namely, without alteration of Peyer's patches, — should never be observed in Paris, where fever is so frequent. [7] M. Louis states in his admirable and elaborate work on Typhoid fever, that in every fatal case of fever he had examined there was special alteration of Peyer's patches: and that this alteration with attendant swelling and softening of the mesenteric glands, was the only constant lesion in those cases; and was never found in the [7] bodies of persons who had died of other acute diseases. [8]

The constancy of this lesion in this form of fever contrasted with the absence of it in all other acute diseases, demonstrates its specific nature and | greatly [added] enhances its importance as a character. [9] The | large [added] experience of M. Chomel and subsequent experience of M. Louis has furnished no exception to this two-fold proposition, but accumulated a vast number of facts in its support. [10]

The experience of physicians in this country is widely different | from that of the French [added]. Dr. J. Reid in an accurate and excellent report on Epidemic Fever in Edinburgh, [11] informs us that of 41

---

6. † There are cases of scarlatina without eruption and of measles without catarrah but these cases communicate again the regular type & never occur in epidemics, but merely in isolated cases.

7. (2) This appears to be the case in Boston also in the United States.

8. [P. C. A. Louis, *Recherches anatomiques, pathologiques et thérapeutiques sur la maladie connue sous les noms de gastro-entérite, fièvre putride, etc.*, 2 vols. (Paris, 1829).]

9. † makes it as specific a character as is erupn in sm.pox —

10. [A. F. Chomel, *Leçons de clinique médicale faites a l'Hôtel Dieu de Paris* (Fièvre typhoïde), ed. J. L. Genest (Paris, 1834).]

11. (3) Edinburgh Med: &, Surg: Journal: Oct. 1839
[Henderson and Reid, "Report on the Epidemic Fever of Edinburgh."]

cases in which the abdominal organs were examined after death from
fever, there were two only in which this special alteration of [8] Peyer's
follicles existed: [12] in the same two and in those only, the mesenteric
glands were enlarged and softened. Now the average duration of the
disease before death in these | 41 [added] cases was about 12 1/2 days: a
period at which the alteration of Peyer's follicles in fever is fully characterized, as may be seen by consulting the chapter on deaths between the
8th and 12th days in Louis' first volume [13] — in these 41 cases the earliest
death occurred on the sixth, the latest on the 22nd day.

The same absence of special affection of the intestines was observed
by Dr. Alison in the Epidemic of 1826.[14] He states that in a few cases the
glands of Peyer and Brunner were more [9] distinct than usual but not
more so than he had seen in persons who did not die of fever, or of any
abdominal disease. Of 25 cases in which the abdominal organs were
examined there was one only in which any ulceration could be detected
in the mucous membrane of the small intestines and in that one a single
small ulcer only could be found.

Similar observations have been made in London and in Dublin.

Thus while in Paris fever is always attended with a certain specific
and important lesion [15]; in London, Dublin and Edinburgh that lesion is
absent in a large proportion of cases. Some have attempted to explain
this difference, by reference to the difference of climate, to national
peculiarities in diet, and to other conditions still more vague and indefinite. [10] But this explanation which is entirely hypothetical, and unsupported by analogy, receives a direct negative from the fact, that while the
English are no less susceptible than the French of that form of fever
attended with special alteration of the intestinal follicles, the latter are
not less liable than the former to that other form in which this alteration
is absent, as was proved by an epidemic of that form which broke out
some years ago in the port of Toulon.[16]

The fact that the form of fever in which that lesion is absent, is never
observed in Paris certainly gives | gives therefore [alternative wording] a

12. (4) It is proper to remark that the subject of one of these cases had left Ireland only 11 days
previous to his admission into the Infirmary of Edinburgh and that he was ailing at that time.

13. [Louis, *Recherches*.]

14. [Alison, "Observations on the epidemic fever."]

15. † of the same value as a character with the exanthemata on the epidermal surface [an insert
marked "facing p. 9" is also present and reads "the ulcer-of bowels the same relation to the cause
as the throat to scarlet fever, etc."]

16. † In the epidemic referred to the fever {was not attended with any special lesion of the intes-
tines} exhibited the measles like eruption which characterizes the fevers which have prevailed so
much in Scotland, Ireland & in London & was not attended with any special lesion of the intestines.

strong presumption | at least [added] that the form in question is specifically different from [11] the other form. Let us now see how far that presumption is confirmed or invalidated by other considerations.

Although I cannot speak [17] from accurate records, yet I can venture to affirm from my own experience, that in the form of fever without alteration of Peyer's follicles there is much less tendency to ulceration in membranous tissues generally than in the other form of fever. This is particularly the case in regard to the effects of blisters. M. Louis informs us that in severe cases of fever which recovered, the skin on which blisters had been applied was more or less extensively ulcerated 7 or 12 days after application, in one eighth part of the cases and in a still larger proportion in fatal cases; and in his chapter on treatment he urges, as a strong objection to the use of blisters, that they are frequently followed by ulceration and complete destruction [12] of that part of the skin on which they have been applied (pp. 258–517. Vol: II). Although I have seen blisters extensively used in the other form of fever I have seldom or never seen them followed by the effects here described and which are strikingly illustrated by individual cases in M. Louis' work.

A difference closely allied to this is the much less [18] liability in the form of fever without intestinal affection, to sloughing of the breech and other parts which support the body in lying.

In the report by Drs. Henderson and Reid already referred to, gangrenous spots are mentioned as being observed in one case only of nearly 200, whereas M. Louis informs us that among 138 cases which he observed, the sacrum was in many quite denuded by sloughing, and in a considerable number gangrene of more limited extent [19] took place.

In a series of 36 cases of the same form [20] [13] of fever, which have lately fallen under my observation and of which I kept exact record,

17. * Of course, we admit, pro tempore, that the writer's authority is poor for facts. JF [John Forbes]

18. * That they could ever have been taken for the same disease argues agst want of close observn.

19. † Beds

20. † [Two notes inserted and marked "p. 12"]

Typhus des camps & {maladies} fièvre typhoid[e] — L'une des différences peu nombreuses que nous avons observées entre ces deux affections consiste dans la durée, qui est plus longue dans l'affection typhoide que dans le typhus. Ce dernier cesse ordinairement vers [le] 14eme jour, tandis qu'il est très rare que la première se termine avant le 20eme jour.

Une autre différence consiste dans la fréquence avec laquelle on observe dans le typhus les véritables pétéchies, ou taches pourprées, qui, comparativement, sont rares dans la maladie typhoide — Quant à l'exanthème curtané, ou éruption typhoide, il offre les mêmes caractères dans le deux affections; les seules différences sont dans le nombre des taches et dans l'époque de leur apparition — A lieu d'etre bor[nées], . . .

[Chomel, Clinique médicale, p. 336.]

Statements to make in regard to the epidemic — Personal knowledge of the place — & all the

sloughing of the breech took place in two, and was prevented with great difficulty and only by dint of incessant precautions in two others.[21]

This remarkable tendency to ulceration and sloughing is not observed in other acute diseases, and must be regarded therefore as a special effect of typhoid fever. Upon these grounds M. Louis has been led to give it the second rank as a characteristic of the disease. The difference in this particular which I have pointed out as existing between the two forms of fever is therefore one to which considerable weight must be attached.

The next point of difference which claims attention regards the occurrence of true petechiae. These are not only more frequent, but also [14] much more numerous in the form of fever without alteration of Peyer's patches than in the other form.[22]

In both forms there is an exanthematous eruption, but the eruption of one differs from that of the other both in the extent of surface it covers, and the time of appearance.

In the fever without intestinal lesions the eruption is generally so abundant that it is very aptly described as a "measles like" eruption: a term which could never be applied to the rose-colored spots, which, discrete and generally few in number, — often difficult of detection, — are observed in the other form of fever.

The measles like eruption generally appears from the 3rd to the 6th day: the scanty eruption never according[23] [15] to my experience before the 7th and seldom so soon.[24]

---

inhabitants — twice burnt — class of inhabitants — Mary Brealy & school next door — much like contagion [William Budd, "Intestinal fever," *Lancet* 1859, *ii,* 458 refers to case of M. A. B. — at the Female Orphan Asylum, Ashby Hill, near Bristol, where a typhoid epidemic occurred in 1842.]

21. * The same tendency to sloughing in all. TJ [Thomas Jeffreys]

22. (5) See the works of MM. Louis & Chomel on Typhoid Fever.

23. † [Two notes are inserted marked "p. 14"]

Period of incubation — "Mais d'apres quelques observations, j'ai lieu de croire que cette periode n'est jamais plus courte que de 3 jours, et qu'elle ne va pas au-delà de 7." p. 39.

Symptoms — Exanthema — (4eme jour) "Presque dans le même temps, il paraît une rougeur extraordinaire à la superficie du corps, c['est-]a-d[ire] sur l'organe cutané, qui forme l'exanthème."

"My two cases presented the peculiar measles like eruption described by so many authors, which in those cases in which I have been able accurately to note the date of its appearance, first showed itself from the 6th to the eighth day, generally the former — It appeared in one instance on 4th & another time on the 5th day but I never saw it make its first appearance after the eighth" — Ed. Med. Surg. Journ. — West

[The first two quotations are from Johann Valentin von Hildenbrand, *Du typhus contagieux,* trans. J.-Charles Gasc (Paris, 1811), pp. 39, 53; the third is from C. West, "Account of Typhus Exanthematicus in St. Bartholomew's Hospital, London, in 1837-8," *Edin. Med. Surg. J.,* 1838, *50,* 118-45.]

24. * To be enlarged upon. TJ [Thomas Jeffreys]

When I add that the fever without intestinal affection is of shorter duration than the other; — that the febrile movement especially subsides earlier: — that cordials are supported, or, rather, required at an earlier period of its course: — that the average age of persons attacked is greater, — and that the protection conferred by one attack against a recurrence in the same individual, [25] is much less certain than in the fever with intestinal affection; [26] — and lastly that the former rarely or never occurs sporadically, but the latter very frequently, I shall have passed in review all the most important particulars in which these forms of fever differ. [27] Many of them are it must [28] [16] be acknowledged differences of striking import and greater than are observed between recognised varieties of other acute specific diseases. But to counterbalance this, there is it must be acknowledged also, more complete agreement in the symptoms and greater resemblance in the aspect of these two forms of fever than between any two diseases specifically different. [29]

In both forms there is the dusky hue of countenance — the prostration disproportionate to local symptoms — the indifference to surrounding objects — the tendency to drowsiness and stupor — the same character of delirium.

In both also, there are [17] tremors and subsultus tendinum — dry tongue and sordes — impairment of vision — ringing in the ears and deafness — a disposition to repeated epistaxis.

As this group of symptoms gives a striking aspect and renders fever in many cases an object of instant recognition, the agreement of the two forms of fever in regard to them naturally leads us to consider these forms as mere varieties of one disease. The most material point of difference between them | that namely relatg. to the intestinal aff. [added] being hidden from view, interferes but little with the bias this impressive group of symptoms is so apt to produce.

In order however to guard against this bias and to form a correct

25. * Qy. See Essay No. J.F. [John Forbes]

26. [Recall that many of the febrile epidemics known to Budd that did not exhibit the intestinal lesion may have been accounts of relapsing fever epidemics.]

27. (6) For confirmation of these statements compare the results obtained by MM. Louis & Chomel with those by Drs. Henderson & Reid. (Louis sur la Gastroenterite — Chomel, Leçons Cliniques sur la fièvre typhoide.) Edinburgh Med. & Surg. Journal. Oct. 1839. Vol:xviii See also the last Chapter of this Essay.

28. † [A note added to the manuscript and marked "p. 15" reads as follows:]

The proof of these points should accompany their statement. May not the much smaller prevalence of the London fever account for rarity of sporadic cases. I see no other mode of accounting for the fact.

29. (7) I have not brought forward the remarkable difference of the two forms in regard to diarrhea; that symptom being the exponent as it were, of the intestinal lesion, it cannot be fairly used in the discussion.

judgement, we must carefully examine how far these symptoms are entitled to the rank of specific characters and by that rank qualified to decide the question [18] of identity.

Such among them as are common to fever and some other diseases are clearly not entitled to that rank, although from being more frequent in fever they may still have some weight as elements of this question.

Now there are many of them, which, though more constant and more strongly marked in fever, are frequently observed in other acute diseases. Prostration disproportionate to local symptoms; — drowsiness — delirium of peculiar type — dry tongue and sordes, are common to typhoid fever and others of a group of diseases of which the essence consists in contamination of the blood with some principle which by its quality or undue quantity acts as a poison to the system. Of the specific nature of such principle these symptoms give [19] no criterion.

Of that group of diseases, phlebitis | or purulent infectn including puerperal fever [added]; — certain forms of erysipelas — some cases of influenza, — the stage of cholera which succeeds reaction are familiar examples.[30]

Acute inflammation of the lungs or other important organs in the aged is also frequently attended with the same symptoms.

Also is it currently said, that these forms of disease give rise to typhoid symptoms: a phrase which implies the truth of the statement here made.

Tremors and subsultus tendinum although less common (except in idiopathic affections of the nervous centres, which for obvious reasons must be excluded from consideration) are yet observed in many diseases of the group and especially in phlebitis | & erysipelas [added].

Deafness although of [20] much less intrinsic importance, holds a much higher rank as a characteristic, since, unless where the effect of stupor or of special lesion of the organ of hearing, it does not occur in any other acute disease; — at least in such as[31] are observed in this country — This symptom bespeaks, therefore, great specialty of action in the cause of fever.

Impairment of vision, as also repeated epistaxis are observed in many other forms of disease and particularly in influenza.

These symptoms are however very much more common in both forms of fever than in any other acute disease.

It appears therefore that many of the characters in which these forms

---

30. † notice particularly puerperal fever

31. † I believe I am wrong here — It is very common in puerperal fever & {other} purulent infections from other causes — viz. traumatic.

of fever agree, do not upon closer examination fully bear out that impression which at first sight they [21] are so apt to make: but that when tried by the criterion of specific value they lose much of their significance as characteristics, and their weight therefore in the determination of the question before us.

Thus reduced to their legitimate value, it seems to me that they are greatly outweighted by the mass of differences in regard to characters of specific importance (specific because not observed in other diseases) that was brought forward in the first part of this discussion.

The presumption with which we set out, namely, that the form of fever attended with special lesion of the intestinal follicles, is different in species from the other form, has therefore been much strengthened by this comparison of the more striking points of their symptoms and morbid anatomy. Still however we have nothing [22] beyond presumption for it is evident that proof cannot be attained by considerations of this order.

Happily, however, the final determination of this question upon grounds from which there is no appeal, is within the reach of well directed and patient research.

A sure criterion and the only sure one of the specific identity or difference of these two forms of fever is furnished by the faculty, which belongs to both,[32] of propagating[33] by contagion. If these forms be mere varieties of one disease it necessarily follows that one communicates the other: the first term of this proposition involves the second. — It is for those who have opportunities of observation in places where both forms are common to determine, whether or not this be the case. The task is difficult, and requires the [23] accumulation of a great number of facts, and strict accuracy on the part of the observer, but its accomplishment will well repay all the pains that may be taken.[34]

But it seems to me that the answer to this question is in great measure anticipated by what happens in Paris: Surely if that form of fever attended with special alteration of the intestinal follicles were capable of communicating the other form, some instances of that other form would happen among the countless cases of fever, that are every year carefully observed in that city[35] — Yet such is not the case — Is not

32. (8) This will be proved in the sequel.

33. * Is this proved in Essay No ? [Again possibly by Forbes, no initials]

34. (9) It is idle to bring forward as an argument, the fact that when fever is prevalent one half of the cases may exhibit special lesion of the intestines and the other half not; that proves nothing more than that both forms of fever may prevail at one season.

35. (10) Some may fancy that M. Louis' chapter on "fièvre typhoide simulée" may contain cases of this form of fever. That is not so, as the slightest attention to the individual cases will satisfy anyone.

the inference almost [24] certain that the form of fever with special lesion of the intestines does not communicate the other form? Thus every new point of view gives strength to the presumption that these forms of fever are different not merely in type but in species.

Whether future research shall improve this presumption into a certainty or on the contrary show it to be groundless, we are at present bound to act under its direction, and in all that relates to these forms of fever, to consider them as different diseases. Such is the course adopted in the following pages. To justify that course is the chief purpose of this chapter. I trust it has not needlessly nor too long detained the reader from the express objects of the Inquiry proposed.[36]

36. * As all the other phenomena are admitted to be similar if not identical in the two fevers e.g. contagion — general aspect — duration — exanthema — I hardly think this postmortem single appearance shd. be allowed to constitute a specific difference. Moreover I expect that the pathognomonic sign admitted by the author (origin of both from one contagion) is to be had. J.F. [John Forbes]

CHAPTER 2ND

Inquiry into the causes and mode of propagation of that form of continued fever which is attended with special alteration of Peyer's follicles.

I have good reason for believing that this is the only form of typhoid fever which occurs in that part of England in which I reside; in rural districts at least.

A considerable number of professional friends well qualified to judge, have informed me that this is the only form of typhoid fever they ever meet with, and I have assured myself by dissections, and by accurate observation of symptoms [1] [26] that it is the only form which ever occurs in my own practice.

This fever is most commonly sporadic, but in some seasons is epidemic in particular localities, affecting a considerable proportion of the population of a given village, for instance, while the inhabitants of neighbouring villages may remain healthy.

I have lately witnessed an epidemic of this kind in a large village, and as nearly all the cases were under my own care, I was enabled to ascertain with much exactness all the circumstances attending the outbreak and subsequent spread of the distemper.

A long residence in the same village having made me intimately acquainted with the occupations, habits and family connections of the population, improved my opportunity for investigating the share [27] which intercourse had in propagating the fever.

I took notes of all the observations I made in reference to these points and from those notes I have written the following narrative, which I do not hesitate to introduce here, being well assured that it is to the attentive observation of particular epidemics that we must look for information regarding the causes and mode of propagation of fevers, as indeed of all epidemic diseases.

---

1. †[Note inserted and labeled "p. 25"] Establish the diagnosis of the N.T. epidemic by referring to details — diarrheae — exanthem — experience in Louis's wards rendered me perfectly familiar with its appearance.

The village in which this epidemic happened is twenty miles distant
from the nearest large town, but in pretty active intercourse with it.[2] The
population counts about 1300 and is almost exclusively agricultural; — a
small proportion (chiefly women and children) are employed in a serge
factory. The village has been almost wholly re-built since 1832; having
been nearly destroyed by two fires, which hap- [28] pened, one in 1832
and the other in 1834. Only four of the houses lately visited by fever were
of those that escaped destruction in these two fires. Forty years ago there
was a very fatal epidemic of fever in the village which since that time has
been remarkably free from fever, and much and justly noted for general
salubrity. Within the last ten years there have not been ten cases of fever
in the village, and before the outbreak of the late epidemic, there had not
been a case for nearly a year and a half.[3]

To give further assurance that this epidemic was of that kind of fever
described at the head of this Chapter, I may state that in every case there
was spontaneous diarrhea | as an early symptom [added][4]; profuse in
many; | in many one of the worst symptoms [added] — and that in one
fatal case there were before death unequivocal signs of peritonitis from
perforation of the bowel, and in another which [29] I examined after
death, I found the well known ulceration of Peyer's patches with swelling
of the mesenteric glands, and other characteristic lesions.[5]

The epidemic began in July 1839 with two cases.

Ann Northam aged 16, and Mary Davenish aged 7 began to droop
the 8th July and were both laid up with fever on the 11th; neither of
them could trace any exposure to contagion.

Mary Davenish lived a quarter of a mile from the village in a
detached row of cottages, but she attended a girls' day-school in a small
court across the street from Ann Northam's.

Northam's house and this school are marked A & A' in the accom-
panying map,[6] which was drawn with a view to render the narrative
more clear and intelligible. [Map missing from ms.]

The child Davenish, had never been absent [30] from home and
Northam had not been away for many months: nor had there been any
visitors in the house of either. None of the family of the former had ever

---

2. [Exeter.]

3. * Was not the occurrce of fever, then, proof of some new element?

4. † all this to be enlarged upon

5. * It is to be regretted that only one dissection can be adduced in proof of the position that this
epidemic was Pyerean (or Peyerean?) Typhus [This note is not labeled J. F. but appears to be the
same hand]

6. (*) In face of the title page.

had fever; Northam's father had fever about nine years before, and was the only one of the family that ever had it.

The third attacked was Martha Davenish, aet. 9, sister of Mary Davenish and school and bed-fellow with her.

She was laid up the 2nd August, two days after her sister had become convalescent. She had continued to attend the school during the illness of her sister, as also to sleep with her.

The fourth was a sawyer named Cheriton, who had been lodging some weeks in the house next the school and which is marked, B, on the map.

He began to droop on the 26th July. On the 2nd August he returned to his own home, nine miles distant. Two days after his return he [31] was laid up and died after an illness of five weeks. The house in which he lodged in the village was a public bake-house.

The 5th, Thomas Hooper aet. 26, was laid up the 8th August, having been ailing from the 2nd August. At that period Mary Davenish was the only one of the sick out of bed, and she lived at a distance. Hooper had not been in direct intercourse with the fever patients. His house is marked, C, on the map.

The 6th, was a sawyer named Allen and the mate of Cheriton.

Allen also lodged in the house next the school and had slept with Cheriton before the later left the village. The 9th August Allen felt unwell and removed to his own home about nine miles distant. Four days afterwards he was laid up with fever.

I shall have occasion to speak further of these two men.

Between the 16th and 27th August inclusive ten fresh cases occurred; all in [32] different houses; in families in various conditions of life, and for the most part not in habits of intercourse. The houses are numbered in the map, with figures expressing the order in which the cases occurred. Not more than two occurred in any given day.

Thus 13 of the first 16 cases happened in different houses: a fact unfavourable to the supposition that the fever had spread [7] by contagion; for upon that supposition it would have been expected that the disease would first have been communicated to the families of the sick, especially as the sequel proved in many cases that members of these families were susceptible of it.

---

7. (11) I may here state that throughout this Essay this word contagion is used in its widest sense, as expressing the communication of a given disease through whatever medium, by means of some agent generated within and thrown off from the body of a person infected with such disease.

Up to this period therefore all the appearances were unfavourable to the supposition that the fever had spread by contagion.

The first cases could not be ascribed to that origin without multiplying hypotheses seemingly unwarrantable in the circumstances of the case; for no direct exposure to contagion [33] could be discovered and the previous history of the place rendered the existence of fomites extremely improbable; — the subsequent spread of the fever could not be explained by the agency of contagion without violating all received notions on the subject.

On the contrary all the circumstances seemed to bespeak the agency of some general cause of disease independent of intercourse — such as miasmata, — to which the sick had been exposed in common; and this was also countenanced by the relation which the early cases bore to each other in regard to neighbourhood, as may be seen by a glance at the map.[8]

Two of one family — the Davenishes, had indeed been successively attacked, but this instance was in reality rather favourable than otherwise to the last supposition. It will be remembered [34] that these children lived at a distance from the village, but attended the school opposite Northam's and marked, A', on the map. The rest of the family, who had no occupation in the village, did not take fever, although the mother and an elder sister slept in turns with the children during their illness. No other cases of fever occurred in the adjoining cottages, but it has already been stated that two sawyers who lodged next door to the school which these children attended, were laid up with fever immediately on their return to their own homes. The natural inference from this particular instance was, therefore, that the children by their resort to the village had been exposed to a cause of sickness independent of intercourse, but affecting them in common with the other sick.

I have said that up to this period of the epidemic all the appearances seemed [35] to bespeak the agency of such a cause; I should have made one exception, namely the slow succession of the cases. — Fifty days had elapsed and only 16 cases had occurred; — for the most part in single succession. These cases would therefore have seemed more like the work of contagion than of a cause common to all, if that view had been countenanced by the other circumstances of the case. It is impossible to deny

---

8. (12) To make this appear it is necessary to state that the map includes only the central part of the village. This known, it may be seen that the group of cases referred to affects a certain degree of centralization. The houses in which they occurred are coloured in red.

too that some amount of intercourse, direct or mediate, had taken place between the subjects of these cases in so considerable a lapse of time.

I can indeed mention one instance in which a case of fever might with some plausibility be ascribed to contagion received from mediate intercourse with the sick.

The subject of the 10th case was one of my brothers, aged 20; he had not been near any of the sick, but I was then much engaged in attending [36] upon them, and also was a good deal in company with my brother.[9]

Parallel instances might have occurred and have passed unnoticed.

In estimating the lapse of time as evidence in favour of the supposition that the sickness had spread by contagion it must be borne in mind, that, generally, the germ of fever is received into the system a considerable time before any symptoms of illness appear.[10] Facts will be related in this chapter which seem to shew that this interval, — commonly called the latent period, — often occupies from ten to fourteen days.

Applying the indication derived from these facts to the particular cases of this epidemic, we must, in order to arrive at the probable moment at which the germ of sickness was received in each case, count back 10 or 14 days from the first symptoms: — a [37] calculation which materially reduces the amount of intercourse that might have been concerned in the propagation of the fever and which brings the moment of reception of the germ in many of the earlier cases so near to that of illness in the first cases, that the chances that these latter had transmitted that germ to the former by <u>mediate</u> intercourse are greatly diminished.

If this reasoning were admitted, the early cases of this epidemic would furnish evidence of a positive rather than negative character in favour of the miasmatic origin of fever. For if a single case offer only negative evidence; arising from our inability to trace such case to a source of contagion; on the other hand, a number of cases, occurring in a group, and in such order as to preclude the possibility of one being the cause of the others, furnishes evidence of a positive character indicating some cause such as miasmata common to[11] [38] all the cases of the group.

9. [Thomas Septimus Budd.]

10. [*Germ* was used from the eighteenth century as a word meaning "that from which anything springs or may spring," while it began to be used medically early in the nineteenth century meaning "vaguely, the 'seed' of a disease." *Oxford English Dictionary* s.v. "germ."]

11. †[Insert marked "p. 37"] In an Article which lately appeared in a leading journal Dr. Camps' account of the Cowbridge fever is made the subject of very trenchant ridicule. But this is, surely, not quite fair. If I mistake not, this gentleman went to Cowbridge in the service of the

But the fundamental step in this reasoning the time namely, assigned to the latent period is not sufficiently sure to serve as foundation

---

General Board of Health, and a glance at the proceedings of that Body will show that in giving the results of his inquiries he faithfully reflected the views of his employer.

To have finally superseded — in the case of typhoid fever — the doctrine of contagion by the theory which attributes the disease to the gases evolved by the decay or putrescence of all sorts of organic substances was long considered the highest scientific triumph of the Board in question.

So that Dr. Camps' report was not only in harmony with the "sanitary science" of the day, but with what were supposed at that time to be the most advanced views upon it.

In proof of this I may cite another fact which is still more conclusive. In 1858, five years after Dr. Camps had communicated his report to the Epidemiological Society, Dr. Murchison, — a physician whom in this matter, will be allowed to be a preeminently representative man — published in the Medico-Chirurgical Transactions a very interesting and elaborate Essay on the "Etiology of Continued Fever."

In this Essay the Section on typhoid fever opens with the following passage —

"I have already shown that the causes of typhoid, whatever they may be, differ from those of typhus, in being for the most part of a very limited and circumscribed character. What these causes really are I shall endeavour to explain under the following head: Putrid emanations from decomposing organic matter in Drains, Cesspools, Churchyards &c. and organic impurities in drinking water." Now the best possible proof that Dr. Camps' version of the Cowbridge fever did not do violence to current medical opinion is the fact that an abstract of it was introduced by Dr. Murchison without note or comment in the section thus headed, among the illustrations of his general theorem.

{But perhaps the following illustration from the same section puts the matter in a still stronger light} [Illustration not given]

The account of this outbreak with which the present chapter opens is, in fact, reprinted almost verbatim from Dr. Murchison's words.

But perhaps the following illustrations from the same section of Dr. Murchison's Essay puts the matter in a still stronger light.

In the same chapter and under the same heading with the Cowbridge case this distinguished writer cites the following case.

> In the first vol. of the "Transactions of the French Royal Academy of Medicine" an outbreak of fever which occurred in 1747 among the girls of the Maison d'Enfant Jesus is recorded. It was generally admitted to have resulted from the disgusting effluvia which proceeded from an adjoining field, in which a number of cattle had been buried, scarcely beneath the surface of the earth. That the fever was typhoid there seems little doubt from the following symptoms which characterized it, viz: fever with great prostration, tympanitis, abdominal pain, diarrhoea, and sudamina. Thirty of the girls were seized all at once, shortly after the interment of the cattle. (MedicoChirurgical Transactions — Vol. XLI. p. 264)

The whole of this section of Dr. Murchison's Essay is, in the highest degree worth studying, as illustrating the views as to the cause of typhoid fever in fashion at the time of its publication. To assert or suggest a genetic connection between the effluvia from dead oxen and typhoid fever is at least as remote from present views as to ascribe it to emanations from stables and stagnant rain water.

Having quoted Dr. Murchison it would be wrong not to add that in the work on fever which he has since published and of which the paper in the Medico-Chirurgical Transactions was the precursor, he appears to have very materially modified his views.

In the chapter on the cause of typhoid fever in the book, the dead oxen, the churchyards, the stables, "et hoc genus omne" are all dropped out — and the illustrations are restricted to cases in which fever is supposed to have been caused by contamination of air and drinking water by (human) sewage.

The Cowbridge case is indeed retained but the following footnote is appended to it.

"This case is here cited more to show the local origin of the disease than as demonstrating its connection with organic impurities."

Between the date of the publication of the Paper in 1858 and that of the Book in 1862, the true

for a weighty argument. I shall show it to be probable that this time is in reality very variable.[12]

But the force of negative evidence increases with every particular instance and may become considerable when these are numerous.

I have already remarked, incidentally, that this form of fever is most commonly sporadic in the country.

As epidemics are rare, the sporadic cases on the long run outnumber the epidemic ones. Of the great number of sporadic cases that fall under my observation there are many that cannot be traced to direct origin in contagion, and not a few in which such origin [39] seems improbable.

The foregoing facts, taken together, contain that order of evidence which is usually admitted as proof of the origin of fever in miasmata or some cause independent of contagion. I do not know that stronger evidence of that origin has been anywhere advanced.[13] In order however

---

history of the Cowbridge fever had become very generally known, and a great part of the evidence bearing on the propagation of typhoid adduced in these pages had been published.

{Is it too much to assume that this evidence had rendered the stable theory palpably untenable}

Whether this last circumstance had anything to do with the insertion of the footnote I have not the means of knowing.

However this may be I cannot but think it a very significant fact in relation to the doctrine advocated in these pages, that Dr. Murchison — if I read him rightly — now places the cause of typhoid fever exclusively in <u>excreta</u> from the human intestine.

It is but one step more to admit that these excreta, in order to produce this fever, must be the actual offspring of it.

[I have not been able to identify the "Article which lately appeared in a leading journal" that subjected Dr. Camps to "trenchant ridicule." Dr. Murchison's book is Charles Murchison, *A Treatise on the Continued Fevers of Great Britain* (London, 1862); Dr. Murchison's paper was "Contributions to the Etiology of Continued Fevers, . . ." *Med.-chir. Trans.*, 1858, *41*, 219-306. Dr. Camps originally read his paper to the Epidemiological Society in March 1855, "On the Occurrence of Fever at Cowbridge, Glamorganshire, South Wales, in the Autumn of 1853," which was abstracted in several journals, the most available of which was the *Lancet*, 1855, *i*, 460. Dr. Camps' report was secondhand; he visited Cowbridge for the General Board of Health in 1854.]

12. † modify language

13. (13) That is, evidence of accurate kind. There is a great plenty of broad and sweeping assertions unsupported by accurate evidence, but with these I have nothing to do. Thus it has been stated by a writer of great authority that in the epidemic of 1817 in Ireland, fever sprang up in all parts of the island at once, and "Appeared like a shock at each extremity of the Island." — anyone who will look over the Reports of the Parliamentary Committee of Inquiry on Contagious Fever in Ireland or the Returns from different hospitals in the work of Barker and Cheyne, may easily convince himself of the extreme inaccuracy of this statement. It plainly appears from those Reports, that the spread of the disease was, as far as time was concerned, exactly like that of other contagious diseases. The complete exemption from fever through the whole course of the epidemic of the islands of Rathlin and Cape Clear, the inhabitants of which gave up all intercourse with the mainland, plainly shows that something more than the common causes of sickness was needed for production of the disease. (See Barker & Cheyne vol:i p:98.99) [F. Barker and J. Cheyne, *An Account of the Rise, Progress, and Decline of the Fever Lately Epidemical in Ireland,* 2 vols. (Dublin, 1821) 1, 98-99.]

Nothing tends so much to embarass inquiry as the very reprehensible practice of indulging in general and sweeping assertions in regard to a subject the investigation of which, on account of its great and peculiar difficulties has need of caution and accuracy at every step.

to interpret these facts rightly, it will be necessary to inquire whether or not analogous facts be observed in connexion with diseases generally acknowledged to have contagion for sole origin; smallpox namely; measles and scarlatina.

I have not in my possession, nor have I been able to find in authors, accounts stating the exact order in regard to dates and neighbourhood, of the early cases of any outbreak of smallpox, measles, or scarlatina in villages or small towns.

[40] The want of such narratives is much to be regretted since if faithfully written, they could not fail to throw much light on the question before us.

If I may be permitted to state an impression derived from recollection, it is, that the early cases in particular epidemics of these diseases are far from uniformly following that order which we should have supposed to be the natural order of propagation by contagion, but that they are often scattered in separate houses much after the manner of the early cases of the epidemic of fever of which I have given some account.[14]

It is quite certain also, and must be well known to experienced practitioners, that cases of smallpox, scarlatina, and measles, frequently occur which cannot be traced to any source of contagion. Dr. Gregory states indeed "that of the numerous cases received into the smallpox hospital, not one in twenty is ever able [41] to trace the disease to any source of infection, but it is believed to arise from cold, fatigue, change of air, or some similar circumstance." (Cholera Gazette N.2).[15] Elsewhere, he remarks that "great difficulties are experienced in tracing the source of contagion in numberless cases, and that the doctrine of spontaneous origin admits of being supported by some ingenious and plausible arguments." (Cyclopedia of Pract: Medicine, art: S:pox)[16]

The smallpox entirely disappeared from Boston in New England at 7 different times and each time for intervals of many years. In 3 only of these instances could the channel of its re-introduction be discovered. But Dr. Henry justly remarks "that these three instances render it much more probable that the poison causing the disease should in the remaining four have been imported anew than that it should be again generated. For though | — he adds [added] it cannot be denied that a poison

14. *I assent to this J.F. [John Forbes] Doubtless J.C. [John Conolly]

15. [George Gregory, "Essay on the Periods of Incubation of the Various Morbific Germs: Addressed to the Central Board of Health," *Cholera Gazette*, 1832, *1*, 54-64.]

16. [George Gregory, "Smallpox," in John Forbes, Alexander Tweedie, and John Conolly, eds. *The Cyclopedia of Practical Medicine*, 4 vols. (London, 1833-35), 3, 735-51, p. 743. Budd has changed the emphasis from "spontaneous" in the original to "numberless."]

may be again [42] elaborated by a concurrence of the circumstances which originally produced it, yet in assigning causes we must be guarded [*sic,* guided] by actual observations not by possible contingencies." (Report of the British Associatn. 1834) [17]

In the Report just quoted Dr. Henry relates, on the authority of Dr. Roget, the case of a prisoner at the Millbank Penitentiary, who was seized with smallpox notwithstanding his apparently perfect insulation.

I have, myself, knowledge of a case of smallpox which it was impossible to trace to a source of contagion. It happened in the village in which I reside, — and at the time it occurred there was no other case in the whole neighbourhood, nor was smallpox prevalent anywhere in the county.

Instances of measles and scarlatina not traceable to contagion are still more common; — so common indeed that particular examples are [43] seldom put on record but writers are content with stating the general fact.

Dr. J. Clark in his narrative of the epidemic of scarlatina that visited Newcastle in 1780 states that the introduction of the disease into that town could not be discovered. (Dr. J. Clark on Fever, p. 24). [18]

In Bateman and Willan's reports of the diseases of London, [19] at p. 263, I find the following interesting record. "1815 Spring — the eruptive fevers appear also to have occurred only sporadically, and even in very close courts in which we witnessed them, to have shown no considerable tendency to spread beyond the families in which they appeared." p. 263

The sporadic occurrence of measles and scarlatina is noticed in all treatises on these disorders.

It appears from these statements that circumstances exactly similar to those [44] which have been considered to indicate for fever an origin independent of contagion, are also observed in connexion with smallpox, scarlatina, and measles; diseases almost universally believed to originate in contagion alone.

It appears that a great number of cases of these diseases occur which cannot be traced to a source of contagion, and that it is often so with the first cases of particular epidemics; also, that some cases arise in situations that seem perfectly isolated, and that sporadic cases of these diseases are by no means uncommon.

17. [W. Henry, "Report on the State of Our Knowledge of the Laws of Contagion," *Report of the Fourth Meeting of the British Association* (London, 1835), pp. 67–94.]

18. [John Clark, *Observations on Fevers* (London, 1780).]

19. [Thomas Bateman, *A Practical Synopsis of Cutaneous Diseases According to the Arrangement of Dr. [Robert] Willan* (London, 1817).]

From this we must infer either that all these contagious diseases have also an origin independent of contagion or that the circumstances just stated; and which are common to them and typhoid fever, do not really imply such an origin. I need scarcely say that in the case of smallpox the [20] first inference is quite inadmissible. [45] In the case of measles and scarlatina, few will consider that inference justified by the circumstances just enumerated, of which the main force consists, after all, in evidence of negative character; in our inability, namely, to trace particular cases of each disease to a source of contagion.

The following remarks on this point, by Rasori are so ingenious and apposite that I shall be excused for quoting them. They are taken from his excellent work on petechial fever. [21]

> Let medical observers be willing therefore to begin to distrust, at least the origin of petechial fever in various causes relating to food, locality, atmospheric changes, to everything in short, but contagion: let them consider that this etiological doctrine has in ultimate analysis no other foundation than that of negative facts; that is to say, our inability to see whence comes the contagious fomes that is deposited in the locality of the outbreak — that negative facts carry with them, if not other- [46] wise supported, a strong presumption of fault in the observer, and that this presumption which has been verified so many times in the experimental sciences, is again verified in the most luminous manner in animal physiology in relation to the theory of spontaneous generation, which was so many ages an error

---

20. (14) I need not detail here the paramount considerations which establish the single origin of smallpox and of which that arising in the fact that this disease has never been found in newly-discovered countries is but one among many.

It is idle to talk of the virus of this disease being generated anew by possible concurrence of the circumstances which first produced it. The first origin of smallpox as indeed of syphilis and other purely contagious diseases is a matter beyond the scope of human research and in that respect on a level with the creation of living things.

21. (15) These are Rasori's words

"Gli osservatori medici vogliano dunque incominciare a diffidare per lo meno dell' attribuita origine delle febrii petecchiali alle varie cause tratte dai cibi, dalle località, dalle vicende atmosferiche, da tutto in somma fuorchè dal contagio; considerino che questa dottrina etiologica non ha in ultima analisi altro fondamento se non quello dei fatti negativi, cioè a dire del non aver visto donde provenne il fomite contagioso depositato nel luogo dello sviluppo; che i fatti negativi portano seco, se non hanno altro appoggio, una grave presunzione di colpa dell'osservatore; e che questo avvenimento, il quale si è verificato tante volte nelle scienze sperimentali se è poi verificato nel modo il più luminoso nella fisica animale, sulla pretesa generazione spontanea, che fu per tanti secoli un errore delle scuole, e di cui non havvi il più analogo a quello de' contagi spontanei. P. 231-32.

[Giovanni Rasori, *Storia della febbre petecchiale di Genova nelgi anni 1799 e 1800* (Milano, 1813), p. 232.]

of the schools; an error to which there is none more analogous than that of spontaneous contagions. [22]

Before concluding this parallel between typhoid fever and the eruptive fevers, it is but just to state that sporadic cases of the former are much more frequent, — in the country at least, — than the same order of cases of the eruptive fevers. [23]

The facts therefore that give presumption of spontaneous origin although of the same order for all these diseases are more numerous in the case of typhoid fever than in that of the others. — On the [47] other hand, we should expect that sporadic cases of the eruptive fevers would be much more rare than sporadic cases of typhoid fever, on account of the much greater tendency of those diseases to spread when once originated. [24]

I shall return to the discussion of this question in another part of this Chapter, and meanwhile proceed with the narrative.

Fresh cases of fever continued to arise in families that were not in habits of intercourse with those already ill, but at the same time a new order of facts appeared.

The mother and two sisters of Ann Northam, — the subject of the first case, — were one after another taken with fever. The father and a child two years old were the only members of this family that escaped. The father had had fever [48] before. All these persons slept in one small room.

In a family of six occupying the house numbered 10 on the map the father and mother were the only ones that escaped fever. The four children were laid up in succession: the first on the 19th of August; the second on the 11th of September; the third on the 20th and the fourth on the 22nd of September.

---

22. (16) The frequent occurrence of itch under circumstances having perfectly the semblance of spontaneous origin shows, that in some cases there is more than analogy between the seeming spontaneous origin of animals and of contagious diseases.

23. † [Opposite p. 46] "so to the ordinary face & { } view of experience is many times satisfied by several theories & philosophies; whereas to find the real truth requireth another manner of severity & attention" — Bacon, Advancement of Learning p. 151.

[Francis Bacon, *Of the Profecience and Advancement of Learning,* ed. B. Montage (London, 1840).]

24. † [Without indicating an exact location Budd has added on the back of pages 46 and 47 the following notes:] In arguing against the common belief that decaying woods generate mildew and other fungi, Mr. Knight says —

and the best known and the most valuable species to mankind, of this tribe of plants, the common mushroom, appears as obviously to spring from horse-dung under favourable cir-

Now the next door to this house there was a girls' Day School numerously attended, and although the girls were at school a great part of the day, during the whole course of the epidemic only one of them was attacked with fever, and the case of that one cannot be taken into account because another member of her family was already ill of fever when she took it.

If therefore the fever in the house next the School was the effect of miasmata the entire exemption of the School girls [49] must be considered a remarkable circumstance, and at least furnished a presumption that the cause of sickness, whatever it might be, was in the interior of the dwelling.

The same remarks apply to the case of the Northams for two doors from them a numerous family remained entirely free from fever.

In a third instance three of one family: — two sons and their mother, — were successively attacked: one on the 22nd August; the next on the 5th September and the 3rd on the 23rd of the same month. The subject of the third case was the mother. She was sixty years old and on that account, probably less disposed to fever than several young persons in the same house who escaped; but she had been the constant nurse of her sons and very watchful over them, allowing no fear of contagion to interfere with the affectionate discharge of her duties.

[50] These facts, however, furnished nothing more than presumption of the agency of contagion; but proof of that agency was soon given by facts of another kind.

It will be remembered that the subject of the fourth case, a sawyer, removed to his own home, nine miles off, soon after he began to droop. Two days after his return home he was laid up with fever of which he died at the end of 5 weeks.[25] Ten days after his death, his two children

---

cumstances as any species of the same tribe appears to spring from decomposing wood, without the previous presence of seeds.† Yet it can scarcely be contended that any vital powers, capable of arranging the delicate organization of a mushroom, can exist in a horse-dung, and the admission of any such powers would surely lead to the most extravagant conclusions. For if a mass of horse-dung can generate a mushroom it can scarcely be denied that a mass of animal matter, an old cheese may generate a mite; and if the organs of a mite can be thus formed, there would be little difficulty in believing that a larger mass of decomposing animal matter might generate an elephant, or a man. Knight. Horticultural Papers p. 204 [-205]

† See Nichol's Forcing, Fruits & Kitchen Gardener.

[Thomas Andrew Knight, *A Selection from the Physiological and Horticultural Papers, Published in the Transactions of the Royal Horticultural Societies* (London, 1841). Walter Nichol, *The Forcing, Fruit, and Kitchen Gardener*, 4th ed. (Edinburgh, 1809). Nichol's was Thomas Knight's reference, quoted by Budd; Knight cited p. 119.]

25. * See Essay No. 3 TJ [Thomas Jeffreys]

were also laid up with fever and both had it severely. The widow continued well. I did not ascertain whether she had ever had fever.

Now at this time there was only one instance of fever in the neighborhood of this man's dwelling, and the history of that instance was much like that just related — It was this, — A young man who lived as farm servant, nearly 20 miles off,[26] [51] was attacked with fever during the convalescence of his mistress, who had been ill of it. He was removed to his own home while in the early stage of fever. He was a long time ill, and before he was convalescent two of his sisters, living at home, were attacked with the same fever.

The case of the other sawyer (the sixth of the epidemic) who left the village when he felt the first symptoms of fever and went through the disease at his own home nearly nine miles off is still more instructive.

A friend who visited this man when he was at his worst, and was called upon to assist in raising him in the bed, was when engaged in this act quite overpowered with the smell from the patient's body, and at the same moment was firmly impressed with a belief that he had caught the fever. He was from that [52] time harassed by continuance of the same smell, and at the end of 10 days was seized with rigor which was followed by typhoid fever of long duration.

This person now became a new source of contagion. Before he was convalescent, two of his children were laid up with fever, and also a brother, living at some distance, but who had repeatedly visited him.

The houses occupied by these three men who were thus successively attacked, were at considerable distances from one another, and there were no other cases of fever in the neighborhood. Only two persons lived in the same house with the sawyer; a man and his wife, — both aged, — and these did not take the disease.

In the course of this epidemic two other persons left the village, when they were in the first stage of fever, and both commu- [53] nicated the

26. † The figure may be used literally here —

2 men who cannot see beyond their nose —

Another fact in the natl. history of the fever — some weeks elapse before 2d crop by the most rigid inductn. — from known facts

— from these two — contagion barely possible

— but although out {of} sight [it] does not necessarily follow that its course ended — is somewhere being contnd. — as faulty

[Reverse of page]

[illegible]

not if the liquid into —

[illegible] which suspended —

in water — much already in a state — of find subdivision

disease to one inmate or more of the houses in which they were afterwards laid up.

The subject of the 14th case, when already ailing, removed to a farm
house eight miles away. Two days afterwards she took her bed, and kept
it several weeks. About ten days after her convalescence the mistress of
the farm fell ill of fever of which she died at the end of five weeks. A few
days before her death, her husband who had been very watchful over
her, was also attacked with fever and is not yet recovered. There were no
cases of fever in the neighbourhood of the farm.

In the other instance the patient who propagated the disease did not
remove to so great a distance. He was a shoemaker's apprentice and fell
ill of fever while his mistress was convalescent of it. He was removed,
[54] in the early stage of the fever, to a small hamlet half a mile from the
village. He was ill four weeks and soon after he became convalescent his
sister two and a half years old was attacked with fever. There had been
no fever in any other house in the hamlet.[27]

These facts scarcely require a commentary. They fulfil every condition of evidence and contain incontrovertible proof of the propagation of
this fever by contagion. They cannot be explained upon any other supposition. The only other explanation that can be offered is, that the illness of all these persons was the effect of some cause, which by a singular
coincidence arose about the same time, in such distant localities, and
happened to affect these persons in succession without the circumstance
of their having approached each other being any wise concerned in [55]
the spread of the distemper among them. But this explanation is built on
a tissue of groundless assumptions, the bare statement of which is their
best refutation.[28]

---

27. (17) From several of these cases, especially those of the sawyers, it would appear that the
latent period of this fever is usually ten days at least.

There is no doubt however that its duration is subject to great variation: — variation contingent
on a number of conditions, of which the principal one seems to be the amount of virus received by
the system. All this is well exemplified for the other form of fever by the series of cases given in an
admirable paper on the subject by Dr. Marsh, (in the 4th Vol: of the Dublin Hospital Reports)
[H. Marsh, "Observations on the Origin and Latent Period of Fever," *Dublin Hosp. Rep.*, 1827,
4, 454–536.]
and in many of which it was quite evident that the disease followed immediately on reception of
the virus.

There is further analogy in the case of smallpox and also, though more remote, in the case of
marsh fevers. I have now before me a case of smallpox caught by single exposure in which the
latent period was extended to 5 weeks. The great variation of the latent period of marsh fevers is
well known.*

* Dr. Haygarth said 30 days TJ [Thomas Jeffreys]
28. † alter language

I might easily multiply instances, from my own experience, of this fever being imported into healthy districts and there propagated, by persons who had contracted it in other places. Such instances are often observed in the country, but I prefer borrowing from M. Bretonneau an example of which this mode of propagation was observed on a large scale. Although the facts occurred in a foreign country, yet the perfect identity of the disease to which they relate with that of which I am now discussing the mode of propagation renders them available to my purpose.

> In 1826 many students of the Military [56] School of la Fleche (Tours) were attacked with typhoid fever which was at that time prevalent in the town. Four died and the anatomical characters of the disease | the specific lesion, namely, of Peyer's patches [added] were carefully ascertained. [. . .] The school broke up earlier than usual, but not before sixty had been attacked with fever. [. . .] Twenty-nine students fell ill of it on their return home and of these twenty-nine eight communicated the disease to some of their attendants.[29]

To consider this as the work of chance would be perfectly irrational, so that these facts leave no resource to the theorist who attributes fever to malaria exclusively.

This series of facts is sufficient for my immediate purpose. It proves beyond dispute that the fever attended with special alteration of Peyer's follicles,[30] (to which, exclusively, the facts relate) is com- [57] municable by contagion. I shall not therefore bring forward the cumulative proof that might be furnished by a greater number and greater variety of facts. Those already adduced contain the highest order of proof which the

---

29. [There is no closing quotation mark in the manuscript, although there should be one at this point. The quotation and translation are very imprecise. Bretonneau wrote: "En 1826, plusieurs élèves de l'école militaire de la Flèche sont affectés en même temps de la dothinentérie, qui règne épidémiquement dans la ville. Quatre élèves succombent, et les caractères anatomiques de l'exanthème pustuleux se montrent dans chacune des recherches nécroscopiques faites avec soin par le docteur Renou. Un des maîtres, originaire de Tours, se rend dans cette ville, et périt, à son arrivée, des conséquences d'une perforation dothinentérique de l'iléon. Réuni à plusieurs de mes confrères, je constate la nature des lésions morbides. Sur ces entrefaites, le général Danliou, gouverneur de l'école militaire, hâte l'époque des vacances; malgré cette précaution, soixante élèves sont atteints, et une des filles du général succombe; le docteur Renou acquièrt la certitude que vingt-neuf des élèves qui se sont rendus chez leurs parens y ont été gravement affectés de la dothinentérie, et que huit l'ont communiquée." Pierre Bretonneau, "Notice sur la contagion de la dothinentérie," *Arch. Gén. Méd.*, 1829, *21*, 57–78.]

30. * The proof is not positive that this epidemic was Peyerean, as only one dissection was made. JF [John Forbes]

question will admit so long as the agent by which this fever is communicated shall elude direct detection. And indeed were it possible to
render this agent palpable and an object of sense, its reality would not be
more assured thereby, nor its agency more clearly shown than by the
facts here related.

It were useless to occupy space by answering objections that may be
raised upon the consideration of negative facts; relating to cases in which
persons seemingly the most exposed to effluvia from fever patients
nevertheless escape the disease. A truth established upon evidence of
[58] positive kind cannot be upset by negative evidence. Moreover a
similar order of facts might be adduced to disprove the contagious nature
of smallpox!

Regarding therefore the contagious nature of this fever as an
established truth, I shall now consider the consequences that may be
deduced from this truth, and especially the way in which it affects the
question of the miasmatic origin of fever.

The first consequence which this truth involves is, that the communication of this fever is effected by means of a material agent, which
thrown off from the body of an infected person, produces the same
disease in another. This agent is therefore the real and proximate cause
of the disease, just as the virus of smallpox is the real [59] and proximate
cause of that malady.

In the cases of this fever that arise spontaneously, or that seem to do
so, the disease can have no other cause,[31] for in these cases there is the
same train of specific effects as follows the <u>observed</u> operation of this
agent, in cases communicated by contagion; including the wonderful
faculty of being further propagated by a fresh evolution of the same
agent.[32]

Nothing implies so certainly the specific nature of a disease, and its
origin in a single, special cause, as this wonderful faculty of being propagated by contagion.[33] But in ignorance of this faculty, we should have
been unavoidably led to the recognition of a specific agent, [60] as cause
of this fever, by considerations founded on its pathology.

---

31. † the same physical cause

32. (*) A facetious friend has remarked that if the agent enters unobserved we at least catch
him as he comes out. [This is one of Budd's original notes; at almost the same location in the
manuscript he later made another note as follows:]

† In both order of cases therefore unity of cause, whatever its origin — necessary to have this
clearly before one.

These cases not less the effect of the typhous virus whatever its origin than cases of smallpox
not traceable to their origin are the effect of the smallpox virus.

33. (18) A faculty which in specific value and in many other points, is so perfectly analogous to
that of generation in living creatures.

The only question therefore, is, whether this agent which observation teaches us, is elaborated by the train of actions constituting the disease, may not also be the product of some other and alien process; as those cases of fever whose origin cannot be traced to an immediate prototype would seem to imply. Those who admit this double origin, for the most part teach that the agent which causes fever, in those cases which cannot be traced to contagion, is supplied by certain miasmata that are evolved in the decomposition of organic matters. It may be urged as an objection 'a priori' to this theory that it is difficult to conceive, that an agent so specific in effects, and which is elaborated in the human body by such a peculiar | train of [added] vital process|es [added] as that constituting a contagious [61] disease, can also be the product of a process so different in nature and carried on in so different a laboratory.

Some have indeed taught that fever miasmata are generated by effluvia from persons in health, but closely crowded in ill-ventilated places; so that according to their theory the laboratory is the same in both origins: the process is however so different that the difficulty is not much lessened.

It has been abundantly shown, moreover, that there is no real foundation for the theory in question so that the objection I have stated remains in force.[34]

[62] I well know that objections 'a priori' have no force when opposed by deductions from experience, but on the other hand such objections, when reasonable and supported by analogy, require as the indispensable condition of their withdrawal that the experience to which they seem opposed, shall be accurate and rightly interpreted.[35]

---

34. (19) Note. It may fairly be alleged that since this objection applies equally to the spontaneous origin of other contagious diseases it must fall if any one of these be proved to originate spontaneously. This is freely granted, but I am not sure that the presumption of such an origin is stronger in the case of any other contagious disease than in that of the fever here considered. Hydrophobia is often cited as a contagious disease of spontaneous origin, but evidence is here so difficult of attainment on every account (the least perplexing of which is the great variety observed in the latent period of the disease) that we cannot admit the double origin of this disease as proved by the imperfect evidence we are yet in possession of.

35. † [Note inserted without notation of exact placement:]
Certain insulated places, such as the island of Rathlin on the coast of Antrim; & that of Cape Clear, on the southern point of {the island} Ireland, were totally exempt from typhus fever, during the period of its prevalence in the rest of the country — In the latter of these islands, instances of common fever occurred arising from heat or cold or too great exertion; but no typhus — The island of C. Clear is 7 miles from the shore & fever was everywhere prevalent along the seacoast adjacent, during the period referred to — Barker & Cheyne — vol:1, p:98-99. [Barker and Cheyne, *An account of the fever*, 1, 98-99.] With regard to the island of Rathlin a curious fact is stated by Dr. M'Donnell of Belfast —

In August 1814 when there was little or no fever on the coast of Antrim, [on going to the island which is about 4 miles from the mainland] I was surprised to find two families, [says the

These reflections naturally lead me back to the facts related in the first part of this chapter. The parallel there drawn between them and a similar order of facts relating to the eruptive fevers tended somewhat to lessen their weight as evidence [63] of the spontaneous origin of fever. In the course of this chapter another order of facts will be developed tending further to the same effect.

I shall relate some curious instances of the propagation of contagious diseases by means that would have escaped detection under ordinary circumstances and I shall shew that, contagious effluvia must be harboured in latent but effective form, and with provision for their secret diffusion, so long as measures accomplishing their extinction shall be neglected by a large portion of the community.

In effect of this, cases of fever must frequently occur seeming to be spontaneous although really originating in contagion, and this consideration would seem to furnish us with a ready and natural explanation of the facts stated in the first part of this chapter, without need of recourse to the theory of spontaneous origin.

[64] Having shown this theory to be open to plausible objections we should be the more disposed to adopt the explanation in question. But does this explanation apply to all the circumstances of the case? Can all the facts here referred to, be thus explained, or do they not still necessitate the conclusion that the agent which produces fever may in some cases be generated otherwise than by that train of actions which constitutes the disease?

Doctor] about the centre of the island with [sic, in] typhus — In the first house I enquired in vain as to the origin of the fever; but on visiting the 2nd house, I discovered that some of the connexions of the family had died in Greenock; they had gone there to visit the sick, and had brought home the clothes of those who had died [at Greenock] in a chest and had taken this disorder soon after their return —

Stokes on contagion — p. 60-61.

[Whitley Stokes, *Observations on Contagion*, 2d ed. (Dublin, 1818).]

By proper treatment & precautions, the disease soon ceased but not until several {had died} were affected & 3 or 4 had died — Since that period & during the whole of the late epidemic, no case of typhus whatever has occurred on that island, although it was very prevalent on every part of the coast opposite Rathlin.

Now it cannot be said [— observes Dr. M'Donnell] — that the exemption of this island arises from the inhabitants being of a different description, being less exposed to cold, heat, fatigue, hunger, bad food, filth, moisture, confined air, and the long list of causes supposed to [sic] capable of producing this dreadful distemper — Their exemption arises from the perfect conviction the people now have that the distemper is portable and that it was imported in 1814.

They send away all itinerant mendicants coming over from Ireland or Scotland; & when a native of the island in November last crossed {over} the channel to attend a relative in fever {they would not allow him} she was not suffered to return —
rigid system of Quarantine

When I shall have gone through all the evidence bearing upon the case, I believe it will be admitted that it is impossible to answer this question in the present state of knowledge.

Already in this discussion powerful motives have appeared for suspension of our judgement; for if the facts stated in the first part of this chapter shew it bold in any one to deny that fever has a spontaneous origin, the considerations [65] since developed show it perhaps equally bold to affirm this.

Having due regard to the abstruse nature of this question, — to the extreme subtlety of the agent concerned, and proportionate difficulty of obtaining certain knowledge of its properties, we are bound to withhold our assent from any conclusion that is not founded upon the most accurate and decisive evidence.

This evidence must be sought for in the exact and well instituted observation of particular epidemics. It cannot be drawn from any other source. If fever really have an origin independent of contagion, facts giving positive and express indication of such origin, and incapable of explanation on any other supposition, are certain to be disclosed by this method of observation.

The comparative study of epidemics of the eruptive fevers will [66] be especially needful to the interpretation of these facts, and will tend admirably to {the} elucidation of the whole question.[36]

The final solution of this question concerns human welfare more nearly than at first appears. For the doctrine of spontaneous origin, if erroneous, gives a false direction to research, and withdraws attention from practical measures necessary for the extinction of contagion, the neglect or enforcement of which cannot be indifferent to mankind.

Having shown that there is yet no assured proof of the spontaneous origin of fever it would be | seems [alternate wording] futile to inquire in what source other than the infected [67] body the agent which causes fever may possible have birth.

Manifold are the circumstances connected with the habits and necessities of man, to which, with nearly equal plausibility, the production of this agent (or in less explicit terms, the spontaneous origin of fever) has in turn and by various observers been ascribed. The variety and frequent incongruity of the circumstances thus assigned to the pro-

---

36. (20) It is very remarkable that this comparative study, which is so full of promise for elucidation of all the dark points in the history of contagion should never have been systematically taken up. I promise myself when opportunity shall offer, to enter this field of inquiry.

duction of an agent so specific in nature, sufficiently testify our [37] real
ignorance of the subject. [38] Dr. Bancroft has, moreover, with great learning and ability shown the inadequacy to this effect of each particular
order in circumstances to which the production of fever has with most
plausibility and with highest sanction been ascribed. [39] The truth of his
deductions in regard to the more important of these circumstances, will
receive frequent illustration in the course [40] [68] of this Essay.

Before proceeding further it will be well to collect, in brief but
explicit form, the leading inferences that are dispersed over the preceed-
ing pages.

They are as follows:

That the frequent occurrence of cases of fever which cannot
be traced to a source of contagion naturally leads to a presumption that this disease may arise spontaneously.

That upon inquiry it is found the same presumption exists for
the eruptive fevers, which are admitted to have contagion for sole
origin.

That this presumption is in all cases open to plausible, though
speculative objections.

That it is, moreover, founded chiefly upon facts of negative
character, and that negative facts may imply nothing more than
deficiency in our means or error in [69] our methods of investigation. [41]

That circumstances relating to the existence of contagious
principles in latent form compel us to allow that these facts may
possibly be explained on the supposition of contagion being the

37. [The manuscript has been altered in pencil to read "testify the real ignorance."
38. † modify
39. [Edward N. Bancroft, *Essay on Yellow Fever, with Observations Concerning Febrile Contagion,
Typhus Fever*, etc. (London, 1811).]
40. † [A note inserted and marked p. 67]
Paris Saturday 17 Feb. [18]55 Times Correspondent —
From the Moniteur "War is not only the crisis in the life of nations it is almost the most decisive
proof of the influence of their manners, of the wisdom of their institutions, and of the elements of
their political and moral greatness. It may be said that the conflict in which France is engaged so
righteously has already exhibited in her armies, in her Government, in her diplomacy, in her
public spirit, in her civilization, those conditions of order, strength, dignity, internal security,
material prosperity, and manly patriotism which enable a great State to undertake all that is just,
to accomplish all that is useful, and to advance towards its object without rashness or feebleness."
[The *Times*, Monday 19 February 1855, p. 9; there is a note that part of the "Foreign Intelligence"
column in which this quotation appears also appeared in the late edition of Saturday which I have
not seen.]
41. † Argumt from analogy of spontaneous genern.

sole origin of fever: although it cannot be shown in our present
state of knowledge, that this explanation will apply to all the circumstances of the case.

That in respect of these various considerations,[42] and of the
abstruse nature of the subject, it is expedient to suspend our
judgement of this question until further research, and the contingencies which time may offer, shall have accumulated more
decisive evidence.

That numerous facts stated in this chapter, which include
every condition of evidence prove that this form of fever is
propagated by contagion.

That this manner of [70] propagation reveals to us the important truth, that a material and specific agent is the essential and
proximate cause of this form of fever, just as the virus of smallpox
is the essential and proximate cause of that malady.

That this inference is as certain for those cases that seem to
originate spontaneously, as for those that can be traced to con-
tagion, and that apart, | from [added] all other considerations,
those founded on the pathology of the disease involve the same
inference.

From this it follows that there is but one efficient cause of this form of
fever, and that cause, a material and specific agent: that all other circumstances are secondary to this, and have no other claim to the title of
cause than in so far as they may increase the activity or favour the diffusion of this agent, or predispose the human body to its operation.

[71] The distinct recognition of this important truth is essential to a
just appreciation and clear arrangement of the circumstances, that may
affect the propagation of this disease, and must be a constant element of
all reasonings on the subject.

Keeping this truth in view we shall avoid the confusion arising from
assigning one and the first rank, as causes, to circumstances of unequal
and inferior importance, and we shall not be misled by appearances so
far as to consider, as real causes of this fever, the more remarkable of the
circumstances among which it may arise.

We shall refuse to admit upon this uncertain | equivocal [alternate
wording] sanction,[43] that this disease may be caused by catching colds,

42. † Modify
43. * In the first place very bold to predicate all this of an agent {whose [illegible] nature}
which is not accessible an object of sense & whose nature wholly unknown to us [no initials but
possibly Jeffreys]

by putrid exhalations, by change of seasons, by want, by crowding of persons in close dwellings, by the use of spoiled provisions, or by any of the various [72] circumstances to which fever has first or last been attributed.

[44] In this matter, not less than in Astronomy, appearances, unless interpreted by the aid of scientific principles | analysis [alternate wording], lead to the most erroneous conclusions.

The secondary importance of many of the circumstances admitted, under learned sanctions, as causes of fever, is indeed often illustrated by the observation of the best writers on the subject. In proof of this statement I may be allowed to quote the following interesting remarks from the Reports on Diseases of London by Bateman and Willan.

> Spring 1808. . . . From the commencement of these Reports [in 1804], we have had occasion to remark the continued freedom from contagious fever which the metropolis enjoys. Since the year 1802 indeed the contagion of typhus has [73] not shown itself to any extent. Yet the seasons have occurred under every variety of temperature, and accompanied with various degrees and vicissitudes of dryness and moisture. In truth from the days of Sydenham downwards, no medical observer has been able to connect any particular epidemic with a specific condition of the atmosphere.
>
> Page 101 [45]

And again: —

> Contagious fever has generally been considered one of the effects of a severe winter, in consequence of the close and unventilated state of the habitations of the poor, which the temperature induces them to resort to for the sake of greater warmth. No such effect however has occurred during this season: the few fevers on the list were mild and not propagated by contagion.
>
> Page 237. [46]

44. † Modify — perhaps expand

45. [Thomas Bateman, *Reports on the Diseases of London, and the State of the Weather, from 1804 to 1816, etc.* (London, 1819), pp. 101-2; "[in 1804]" added by Budd.]

46. [Ibid. The quotation actually reads, "Contagious fever has generally been considered as one of the products of a severe winter, in consequence of the close and unventilated state of the habitations of the poor, which the temperature induces them to resort to for the sake of added warmth. No such effect however has occurred during the present season. The few cases of fever in the preceding list were of a mild type and were not propagated by contagion."]

Again in 1814-15.

To those who recollect [74] the numerous cases of typhoid fevers which called for the relief of Dispensaries [47] twelve or fourteen years ago, and the contagion of which was often with difficulty eradicated from the apartments in which [sic, where] it raged, and even seized the same individuals again, and again, when they escaped its fatal influence, the great freedom from these fevers which now exists even in the most close and filthy alleys in London, is the ground of some surprize. The Fever Institution has doubtless contributed much to the purification of many receptacles of contagion especially within the district superintended by the [sic, this] Dispensary. [. . .] But the diminution of typhus is perhaps too general throughout the Metropolis to be entirely ascribable to [the efforts of] that useful institution. At the same time we cannot observe any contemporaneous progress in the diminution of the causes to which these fevers are usually ascribed, which is at all proportionate to the diminution of fever, [75] or adequate to account for this occurrence: [. . .] — The physicians of dispensaries are well aware that there is still an abundance of dirt, closeness and starvation, immoveably adherent [sic, inherent] in numberless districts which they visit, which appear to be as fully adequate as ever to produce and mature [sic, nurture] the contagion of fevers. [48]

Page 257. [49]

I have already alluded to the work of Dr. Bancroft as containing a full discussion of these topics.

The facts detailed by Parent Duchatelet in his admirable work on the

---

47. † Thus while the circumstances usually assigned to the production of fever are permanent the outbreaks of fever only occasional — testify to the introduction of a new element.

Case of N. Tawton Case of an epidemic in London — Contrast with malaria — marsh fevers [illegible]

48. (21) In the formation of the current opinion that fever is caused by the effluvia of persons crowded in close places, or by putrid exhalations, it is quite plain that the sense of smell has given a bias. That bias is clearly evinced by the language used in reference to this subject by many of the best writers as I could show, if necessary, by numerous quotations. The following pertinent remarks by Brera have application here.

"Souno adunque due diverse materie i contagi, ed i miasmi anco putrefatti Egli è inoltre da riflettersi, che l'odore di putrescenza non costituisce un carattere, che annunzj la presenza del contagio. Le sottilissime molecole contagiose sono ai nostri sensi inodore, nella stessa guisa che prive si ravvisano d'altra sensibile qualità. Il cattivo odore o puzz o può accompagnare i contagi senze che le materie costituenti l'odore entrino a parte de' contagi istessi." Brera de Contagi. Vol. 1, p. 29

[Valeriano Luigi Brera, De'Contagi e della cura de 'loro effetti, Lezioni Medico-pratiche, 2 vols. (Padua, 1819).]

49. [Bateman, Reports, pp. 257-58.]

sewers of Paris are,[50] I think completely subversive of the theory, which ascribes the generation of fever miasmata to the decomposition of organic matters. How can this theory be reconciled with the fact, there averred, [76] that the men whose occupation it is to clean these sewers are remarkably healthy,[51] and that with the exception of instances of untimely death from asphyxia, their life is nowise shortened: — or, with the express declaration, there made, that these men are not subject to putrid diseases! Yet they pass their lives in an atmosphere rife with products of the decomposition of organic matters, to a degree unknown in this upper air, and such as often to cause temporary asphyxia and sometimes, instant death. Moreover in cases of recovery from asphyxia; — a condition testifying absorption to the largest dose of these deleterious principles compatible with life; — the processes which follow are essentially different in nature from[52] [77] from [sic] those of typhoid fever. This is more distinctly shown by the total inability of the sequelae of asphyxia to be propagated by contagion.

In the same work there is an accurate account of many open sewers in Paris, which although a prolific source of noisome effluvia are yet without obvious detriment to the health of the neighbourhood.[53]

The principal foundation for the current opinion that fever is produced by causes, such as are here referred to, is the more frequent outbreak and greater prevalence of this distemper in districts inhabited by

---

50. (22) Essai sur les Cloaques ou Egouts de la Ville de Paris.
[A. J. B. Parent Duchatelet, *Essai sur les cloaques ou égouts de la ville de Paris* (Paris, 1824).]
51. (23) His words are these: ". . . en général, et ceci est digne de remarque, leur santé peut être considérée comme parfait et fort rarement dérangée." p. 122. [see also pp.] 124. 125.
52. † [Facing p. 76 without indication of insertion]

In the appendix to the 4th Report of the Poor Law Commissioners, it is stated by Drs. Arnott, Kay, and S. Smith that the malaria arising from the putrefying animal and vegetable matters produces typhoid fevers. Although I highly respect all these gentlemen, & approve of the practical inferences which they draw from that opinion, so far as it goes, because I have no doubt that vitiated air, like all other causes which weaken the constitution, favour[s] the diffusion of fever — yet I cannot subscribe to their opinion that this cause is of itself adequate to the production of contagious fever. And if trusting to that opinion, the public authorities should think it sufficient, in any situation where contagious fever is prevalent, to remove all <u>dead</u> animal & vegetable matter without attempting to improve the condition of the <u>living</u> inhabitants, I am confident that their labour will be in vain. The true specific cause of the contagious fever, at least of Edinburgh, certainly does not spring from anything external to the living body. I have stated much evidence on this point in a paper in the Edinburgh Medical Journal for 1828 & could easily adduce much more. Alison, Management of the Poor in Scotland p. 11.

[William P. Alison, *Observations on the Management of the Poor in Scotland and Its Effects on the Health of the Great Towns* (Edinburgh, 1840).]
53. (24) See pages 70. 71. 76. 196. op: citat. [Budd later added another note:] † See also p. 18 of the Poor Law Commissioners Reports on the Sanitary condition of the Lower Classes.
[The following is another note inserted and marked "p. 77"]
Parnell's Chemicl. Analys: Qualitatve. — much enlarged — 141 [Edward Andrew Parnell, *Elements of Chemical Analysis, Qualitative and Quantitative*, A new edition (London, 1845)]

the poor, where these causes are also more prevalent.[54] But the partisans of this opinion [78] would have paused before adopting it, had they reflected that exactly the same is observed[55] of the eruptive fevers.[56]

In the course of this chapter there will appear other circumstances relating to the dwellings of the poor, quite sufficient to explain this more frequent outbreak and greater prevalence of fever therein, without reference to these reputed causes.

[79] In deference to these considerations I did not in the narrative with which I opened this chapter make any reference to the state of the drains of the Village where the epidemic of fever which is the subject of that narrative broke out. I may now state that those drains were in as good condition as they have been in, for the last 15 years, whereas, before the late epidemic, fever was uncommonly rare in the Village. By the advantage of situation on a hill side, the drainage of this Village was also much better than that of many neighbouring villages, where however there was no fever, at the time of the epidemic referred to.

From the foregoing considerations it appears, that if this fever have an origin in miasmata, we are at least in complete ignorance of the process by which those miasmata are generated. Thus being [80] unable to recognise any source of this fever-poison other than the human body affected with the disease, all that follows relating immediately to the poison, will of necessity have exclusive reference to that Source.

Having fully assured ourselves that the action of a specific virus is necessary to the production of this fever, we have now to inquire what are the circumstances that render that action effectual.

Will's Giessen Outlines of Qualitatve. Analys: with Tables on Linen — 71 [Heinrich Will, *Outlines of the Course of Qualitative Analysis Followed in the Giessen Laboratory* (London, 1846) a translation of *Anleitung zür qualitativen chemischen Analyse*]

Blue Book — Evidce. on Medl. Reform

On Poisons — By A.S. Taylor — [Alfred Swaine Taylor, *On Poisons in Relation to Medical Jurisprudence and Medicine* (London, 1848)]

54. (25) This is but one of countless instances in the history of medical opinions where the co-existence of two striking facts has been taken to imply the relation of cause and effect between them.

55. †Insert here some numerical Tables by Dr. S. Smith showing that scarlatina is most prevalent in the same metropolitan district in which fever also most prevails — See Appendix to 4th Rept of P.L. Commissioners, pp. 53–54

[Southwood Smith, "Report on Some of the Physical Causes of Sickness and Mortality," Appendix to Great Britain, Poor Law Commissioners, *Fourth Annual Report,* p. 83–94, *PP,* 1837–38, 28, 145 ff.]

56. (26) The objection this reflection contains is well expressed by Brera in the following passage. "Non da effluvi putredinosi, non da vicissitudini atmosferiche anco le più stravaganti e terribili è da ripetersi adunque le cause delle malattie contagiose. Una tale verità rimane oramai

These may relate to the virus itself; — to the persons exposed to its action, — to circumstances touching both the virus and the persons exposed.

In relation to the virus the most important circumstances are the media of transmission and the degree of its concentration.

The most common medium of transmission [81] is undoubtedly the air. There is no need of particular instances to prove this. The notorious fact that fever spreads much more in localities where the air of apartments tenanted by the sick is close and stagnant, than where free ventilation is practised, although the amount of contact and other intercourse be the same, is sufficient proof that the atmosphere is the most common medium of transmission. The same fact plainly shows that, as far as the virus is concerned, concentration is the condition which most certainly ensures its effective operation. Analogy might have led us to anticipate this. Dr. Holland has well remarked that "if we can dilute the matter of small pox, so that it is no longer capable of giving the disease by inoculation equally may the effluvia of certain fevers, capable of communicating the disease in one degree of concentration, be so [82] diluted in other cases, either in their original emission from the sick body, or by distance, or by the state of the atmosphere, that they lose the power of reproducing the disease in its complete and specific form." (Medl: Notes & Reflections, p. 266).[57]

The degree of concentration must depend on the limitation of the atmosphere into which the poison is diffused and the amount of poison supplied.

This last consideration involves all that relates to the condition of the patient furnishing the poison; especially to the period and severity of his illness. As it is quite certain that a much greater quantity of virus is furnished by the case of confluent smallpox than by one in which the pustules are few, we may safely presume that there is more abundant emission of poison in malignant cases of fever than in [83] mild ones. The analogy here is so close that we may draw from it with confidence. But direct evidence to the same effect is not wanting. Dr. Trotter whose

---

[all' evidenza] dimostrata, ed i pochi increduli non saprebbero conciliare come da atmosferiche alterazioni insorger potessero epidemìe vajuolose, tifico-contagiose ec." De Contagi, P. 8. Vol: i.

The same objection applies with equal force to the doctrine that crowding in close apartments is a cause of fever; — and indeed, to almost all the reputed causes of fever. On the inadequacy of putrid effluvia to produce fever, consult also van Swieten's Commentaries on Boerhaave's Aphorisms — No. 1408. [Gerard van Swieten, *The commentaries upon the aphorisms of Dr. Hermann Boerhaave*, 18 vols. (London, 1744–73). There is an additional note opposite this point in the text:] † Expand

57. [Henry Holland, *Medical Notes and Reflections* (London, 1839), p. 266.]

situation as naval physician gave him the best opportunities for investigating all matters relating to contagion, makes the following statement. "We draw the conclusion that a malignant typhus is more apt to generate contagion because we see that slight cases of the same disease, and with mild symptoms do not extend to others, although no means have been used, and in situations too where there was a strong predisposition to assist its action." (Medic:Nautic: p. 175. vol:i)[58]

It is not at all ascertained at what period of the disease emission of the poison commences nor how long such emission continues. In regard to these points direct evidence is wanting, and [84] the indications of analogy are various and uncertain. For practical purposes however it is well to know that fever is seldom communicated to those about the sick when these are removed within the three or four first days of their illness. This has been abundantly proved by the experience of the Navy. It does not follow, however, that emission of the poison does not begin before that period. By similar experience it was ascertained that the spread of small pox in ships was prevented when the sick were removed as soon as the 2nd or 3rd day of eruption, whereas Dr. Gregory[59] states that he has knowledge of facts proving that prior to the eruption and during the premonitory fever the secretions are infectious.[60]

[85] In regard to the period during which, in fever, emission of the poison may continue, evidence is still more deficient. I have knowledge of one instance in which it was quite certain that fever was communicated by a person far advanced in convalescence. To what length of time this power may extend we cannot at present form a probable conjecture. Analogy would perhaps suggest a longer period than is generally thought of. Dr. Blackburn informs us that convalescents from Scarlatina continue to communicate that disease for ten days or even longer after all symptoms have disappeared, and even after desquamation.[61] And Dr. Tweedie states that "he has known in several instances convalescents from Scarlet fever on their removal to a considerable distance from the situation in which they had passed through the disease, infect individuals

---

58. [Thomas Trotter, *Medicina Nautica: An Essay on the Diseases of Seamen*, 3 vols. (London, 1797–1803).]

59. [Gregory, "Smallpox," p. 744.]

60. (26) [*Sic*] In the instance of exanthematous diseases we are probably erroneously led by theoretical notions to connect the first emission of contagious effluvia with the coming out of the rash. It was proved over and over again by cases in the Channel Fleet, that measles are infectious long before this.*

* Qy authority? [No initials, but Forbes]

61. [William Blackburne, *Facts and Observations Concerning the Prevention and Cure of Scarlet Fever; with Some Remarks on the Origin of Acute Contagions in General* (London, 1803).]

[86] with whom they came in immediate contact although many weeks had elapsed from the period of desquamation." (Prac: Cycloped: Medic:)[62]

The determination of these points in regard to typhoid fever — of the period namely: at which emission of the poison begins and ceases — obviously of so much importance to a thorough comprehension of the question of spontaneous origin, can scarcely fail to be accomplished with sufficient precision, if observers be watchful of the opportunities, which the contingencies of human intercourse from time to time offer.

Although this fever is most commonly communicated by effluvia diffused in the air, there is no doubt that porous bodies; — such as tissues,[63] — impregnated with them may also communicate the disease. Some are even of the opinion that effluvia thus imbibed [87] are afterwards emitted in more concentrated and effective form.

Of this manner of communication I may be allowed to give a few examples.

M. Chomel relates an instance that occurred in the Hôtel Dieu of Paris, in which a patient admitted for inflammation of the testicles, and placed in a bed previously occupied by a person ill of typhoid fever, took that disease at the end of a fortnight from admission. M. Recamier has observed two similar instances from the same hospital.[64]

These facts relate specially to the form of fever under present consideration, but if proof of the effectiveness of tainted articles were rested on facts relating to typhoid fevers without distinction of form, that proof would be found in great abundance. It is very distinct in the fact stated by Dr. Tweedie (Clinical Illustrations [88] of Fever p. 88)[65] that the laundresses to the London Fever Hospital, so invariably take fever, that it is extremely difficult to prevail on women to undertake that loathsome office.

This liability of the laundresses of Fever Hospitals, to take fever, is expressly noticed by Dr. Alison also, and has been universally observed in this country.[66]

62. [Alexander Tweedie, "Scarlatina," in John Forbes, et al., *The Cylopaedia of Practical Medicine*, 4 vols. (London, 1833-35), 3, 641-57, although the quotation actually begins, "We have known . . ."]

63. [In the sense of woven cloth.]

64. [Chomel, *Leçons de clinique médicale faites a l'Hôtel Dieu de Paris* (Fièvre typhoïde) ed. J. L. Genest (Paris, 1834), p. 323 cites both his own experience and that of Joseph C. A. Recamier (1774-1852), professor of medicine in the Collège de France and editor of *Revue Médicale*, 1832-38.]

65. [Alexander Tweedie, *Clinical Illustrations of Fever* (London, 1830).]

66. * Not if the linen be put in cold water once or twice. It 'tis said the straw conveys the contagion TJ [Thomas Jeffreys]

The following interesting fact is quoted from Dr. Prichard's work on fever.

> I witnessed this disease in two houses on Redcliffe Parade, where I was the medical attendant, within a short space of time and the cases I allude to occurred in families that were in the habit of frequent intercourse. In one of them a female servant was first attacked and subsequently three children who had been nursed by her. The servant was sent into the infirmary and the family removed into the country while the house [89] was white-washed and as it was supposed thoroughly purified. After their return two female servants were seized with fever and sent into the infirmary: [67] it was found that both these women had slept upon a bed on which the first female who introduced the disease had lain. (Page 36–37).[68]

At page 14 of the report of the Select Committee of Parliament, on Contagious Fever in Ireland, it is related that a person residing at Bally Duff who died of fever had bequeathed his clothes to an inhabitant of the opposite side of the river and soon after this event the disease spread through the family into which the clothes had been received. Numerous instances of the same effect are recorded in the valuable work of Drs. Barker and Cheyne, and in the work of Lind, Pringle, Bateman, Clark, Hildenbrandt [sic] [90] and other eminent physicians; but these already given are sufficient to show that tissues impregnated with the effluvia of fever are very effectual means of propagating the disease.

It is a reasonable belief, and justified by analogy, that impregnation adequate to this effect may be acquired by articles that have never been in actual contact with the sick body.

It is somewhere, related, that smallpox broke out in a family at Liverpool a short time (an interval allowing of the usual period of incubation) after receipt from London of garments that had been made in a room where persons lay ill of smallpox, although contact of these garments with the sick persons had been sedulously avoided. Smallpox was not prevalent in Liverpool when this happened. Dr. Trotter has related [91] a similar but still more remarkable instance. (See p: 300 Medic:nautic: vol:III)

There is also analogy to render it probable that fever may be communicated by effluvia adherent to the clothes of attendants on fever patients, to persons who have not, themselves, approached any one ill of

---

67. † [Opposite p. 89] Sir G. Blane — purifying ships

68. [James Cowles Prichard, *History of the Fever Which Prevailed in Bristol during the Years 1817–19* (London, 1820).]

fever. It is quite certain that the eruptive fevers are sometimes communicated in this way. The following fact is undoubtedly an example of this and is remarkably interesting on account of the limitation of the circumstances. It is quoted from Dr. Trotter's Journal: —

> October 18th. Received a patient in smallpox from the Queen Charlotte. This ship had now been nine weeks at sea, and there could have been no suspicion of the infection having been received directly from any person under the disease. Mr. Murray therefore accounted [92] for it in this manner. The husband of one of our nurses was a soldier on board the Queen Charlotte, and while the patient from the Marlborough in smallpox lay in the Hospital-Ship; this woman had attended him and carried the infection, when she visited her husband about a week before this man sickened. The disease was of the confluent kind; he died on the 4th day.
> (p. 150 Medic:nautic: vol: I)[69]

The following case from the 3rd Volume of the same work is of similar kind.

> The Alcmene frigate [Captain Digby] which sailed from Plymouth three weeks ago, carried out the variolous infection. Two cases first taken ill were confluent and terminated fatally. [. . .] This infection was brought on board by a woman of the town who had buried her child the day before, and died of that disease so that it had been carried in her wearing ap [93] parel. The man who first fell ill messed with this woman and sickened about the 7th day. (p: 103).[70]

I have lately seen two remarkable examples of the propagation of smallpox by mediate intercourse. The first was this: — some children living at a farm, in a secluded spot and two miles from the nearest village were attacked with smallpox. This disease was then prevalent in the village but not nearer. These children had not been near the village nor had any of the smallpox patients been at the farm: but the father and mother of the children had resorted much to the village and to houses where the small- [94] pox was.

The other example being very similar to this I need not relate.

I know also of an instance in which there was every probability from appropriate sequence of events, that a medical man carried Scarlatina

---

69. [Trotter, *Medicina nautica.*]

70. (27) Whoever reads Dr. Trotter's work attentively cannot fail to remark the precise agreement in the circumstances attending the introduction of s[mall]:pox & that of fever into the Channel Fleet.

from a patient ill of it to a family at a distance of many miles and where there were no cases of that disease.

These facts give cause to presume that the following was an example of the communication of typhoid fever by effluvia about the person of a nurse.

The wife of a butcher, in a small town, was attacked with typhoid fever there being no cases at the time in the neighbourhood of her dwelling. She had not been near any person ill of it, but her mother who was a nurse, and who lived in the same house, had, a short time before, been engaged in nursing a whole family ill of typhoid fever and living [71] [95] in a small cottage six miles from this town.

There is every reason to believe, therefore, that typhoid fever, may be communicated by mediate intercourse: Dr. Willan was indeed of opinion, that it is by this means, that fever most frequently finds its way into the houses of the opulent (Lettr. to Dr. Clark).[72]

When many persons ill of fever are crowded in close places, not only various tissues become tainted with contagious effluvia but these effluvia

---

71. † [insert marked "p. 94"] Some years ago a fashionable London physician whose practice was confined to the rich people of the West End gravely assured me that the contagion of typhoid fever was all a myth: that in the course of his time he must have seen hundreds of cases or more and that in no single case had he ever observed anything [to] suggest a suspicion of the disease being of a contagious nature.

It need scarcely be said that the only thing proved by men who reason thus is their own logical incompetence to deal with such questions.

From what has gone before it will be seen at once that the facts in no way justify the inference which this gentleman drew from them. In the well drained mansions the specific excreta of the fever patient are swept away by sanitary appliances before they have had time to develop their latent power. But it would be absurd from this to infer that their function is ended. Harmless as they may appear in the home where first cast forth.

[There is a page of notes missing at this point. These are same sketchy references for the composition "fashionable, large practice, physician in the W. End," etc. on a second sheet] new dwelling they impose on the vulgar, and events which in reality are strict examples of the self-propagation of a contagious fever are set down to the poison which is supposed to be the spontaneous offspring of "sewer gas."

{If the facts are doubly misleading the explanation on the other hand is doubly perfect.} It explains at once the striking immunity in the one | first [alternate wording] case and the fatal liability in the second | other [alternate wording]. It meets completely and equally well the twofold difficulty (Insert to 18 bis.)

Before leaving this topic | the subject [alternate wording] there is one | a [alternate wording] minor question of some importance on which it is well to say a word.

Typhoid fever is a contagious fever propagated by a specific poison as other contagious fevers are. How long after its discharge | it is cast out [alternate wording] from the body does this poison retain its contagious power.

Unhappily there are no data which enable us to return a precise answer to this question. For obvious reasons such data free from ambiguity and bearing upon it must be very hard to get.

{May mention however one or two facts.}

[The notes break off.]

72. [John Clark, *A Collection of Papers Intended to promote an Institution for the Cure and Prevention of Infectious Fevers in Newcastle*, etc., 2 vols. (Newcastle, 1802), 1, 104-5.]

also adhere to the surfaces of more solid materials, in quantity effectual to communicate the disease to such as may afterwards approach them.

Dr. J. Clark of Newcastle states that an instance had been observed by him, in which the contagion of fever had been preserved in one room for two years and infected [96] every new family that came into it.

Numerous facts of similar kind are related by other writers, especially by naval physicians, in whose works they abound. This passing reference to them is sufficient here.

Having passed in review the different forms under which the contagious effluvia of fever may be retained by materials that surround the sick in their dwellings it may now be asked how long these effluvia, thus retained, may continue effectual to communicate the disease. In regard to this we must confess almost entire ignorance. Yet the answer to this question, with some degree of approximation, at least, is absolutely essential to judgement of the question of spontaneous origin.

Lind, Trotter, and Blane, to whose testimony great deference is due, not less on account [97] of their rare sagacity, than of the excellent opportunities they enjoyed for the investigation of this subject were all of opinion that the contagious effluvia of fever harboured by the furniture of ships, may continue effectual in that form for considerable periods of time. [73]

In the absence of all direct facts relating specially to the effluvia of fever I may again be allowed to consult analogy.

It is an assured fact that the liquid poisons — those of smallpox and cowpox — dried at a moderate temperature, — may be kept effective for any length of time, regaining when moistened their infectious properties. Dr. Gregory informs us also that "the clothes and bed clothes of a smallpox patient if closely wrapped up will retain and give out the disease to others at indefinite periods of time." (Cyclop:Prac:Med:) [74]

The following interesting fact related by Hildenbrandt [sic] in his admirable treatise [98] on fever bears still closer analogy to the object of inquiry.

---

73. † [A note is inserted opposite p. 97 on which the smallpox case on the Queen Charlotte was again quoted from T. Trotter, *Medicina Nautica* (n. 58), 1, 150, as on p. 92–93 of the manuscript.]

October 18th. Received a patient in smallpox from the Queen Charlotte. This ship had not been 9 weeks at sea, and there could have been no suspicion of the infection having been received {from} directly from any person under the disease. Mr. Murray therefore accounted for it in this manner: The husband of one of our nurses was a soldier on board the Q. Charlotte; & while the patient from the Marlborough in smallpox lay in the hospital, the woman had attended him & carried the infection when she visited her husband about a week before this man sickened. The disease was of the confluent kind; he died on the 4th day.

74. [Gregory, "Smallpox."]

A black coat which I wore in attending a patient in Scarlatina, and which, without having put it on for more than a year and a half, I wore from Vienna into Podolia, communicated to me, on my arrival, that eruptive disease which afterwards spread from me over that province in which it was previously almost unknown.

(Page 123 French Translation of Hildenbdt.)[75]

Although therefore we cannot determine with certainty and upon sanction of direct facts the limit of the period during which articles tainted with the effluvia of fever may continue efficient to communicate that disease, yet is there every reason to presume that under appropriate conditions and such as must often be realised, this period may be of considerable duration.[76] This presumption is supported by closest analogy, and by the authority of physicians the best qualified by sagacity, and opportun- [99] ity of observation to pass judgement in the matter.[77]

It is impossible not to see how closely these considerations affect the question of spontaneous origin, and how needful is the determination of many most important points before we can approach the discussion of that question with a right understanding of its bearings and with hope of security against the errors into which appearances are so apt to lead us.

Incomplete as these considerations are, and especially, wanting in precision, they yet suffice to show the great importance of fomites as means of the propagation of fever.

From the total neglect by a large portion of the community, — especially by the lower classes in large towns, among whom such extensive epidemics of fever prevail, — of means for the removal or extinction of contagion, a vast amount [100] of contagious effluvia must always be harboured by tissues and various articles that surround the sick in their dwellings.

It is not difficult to see how plentifully this source may provide for

75. [Johann Valentin von Hildenbrand, *Du typhus contagieux*, trans. J.-Charles Gasc (Paris, 1811).]

76. †[Facing p. 98 there is the following note from Thomas Trotter:]
In the course of last summer (1797) four ships of the line had by different means imported sm.pox — The Triumph received it from a woman attending the ship in May at Torbay who came out of {the} a house where the disease prevailed & from her clothes a boy was infected. It appeared just as the fleet was going to sea and Sir A. Gardner ordered a cutter to carry the boy to Plym. Hos. so as to prevent further progress. In August a man sickened on board the Q. Charlotte, & when his case was found to be sm.pox was immediately ordered away by Sir C. Thompson, in Cawsand Bay. p: 120. The captain [Budd has deleted the words "after all" and inserted the apositive "in which . . . spread,"] in which ship the disease spread brought into port 42 men who were unconscious of having had the disease. Before we leave this subject, we beg leave to repeat, that we have always found this contagion completely checked provided the patient is removed before the 3d. day of eruption. p: 123. [Trotter, *Medicina nautica*, 2, 120, 123.]

77. †Analogy of preservation of seeds — of revival of animalcules.

secret dissemination of fever through the community and for the outbreak of this disease under circumstances having the semblance of spontaneous origin — This will receive further illustration in the course of this
chapter.

I shall now recapitulate briefly all these considerations relating to the
virus of fever, with view to determine, more expressly, their practical
bearing on the diffusion of the disease.

It appears first,

That this virus is most commonly transmitted as a cause [101]
of fever, through the air, but that it may also be lodged in effective quantity and form, in tissues and about more solid articles.

That when diffused in the air, concentration of the virus is the
condition which most certainly ensures its specific operation.

That the degree of concentration is proportionate to the amount
of supply of the virus on the one hand, and the closeness of the
atmosphere on the other; and since these conditions are subject to
every possible variation, it is plain that we cannot assign the
sphere of activity of fever effluvia in terms of so many feet, or in
any terms other than such as are expressive of the degree of
concentration.

Dr. Haygarth's attempts to give this the precision of measurement,
although made with laudable purpose, and of assistance in the attainment of a great [102] object, have probably tended to check and
embarass subsequent inquiry.[78]

It is well remarked by Dr. Holland, that: — If a virus can be
transmitted from the body through a few feet of air, we are not
entitled from the partial experiments hitherto made to set any limits
to the extent to which, under favourable circumstances it may be
conveyed through the same or other medium. Common reason here
concurs with the [*sic,* our] actual experience of the transmission of
the virus of certain diseases, in various ways to remote distances.
(Medical notes and Reflections, p. 267)[79]

78. [J. Haygarth, *An Inquiry How to Prevent the Smallpox* (London, 1784).]
79. [Holland, *Medical notes,* pp. 267-68.]
(28) The following fact may facilitate our conception of the transport of minute bodies through
the air to remote distances, with preservation of subtle properties — on some points of the western
coast of France, a lichen is found which is unknown elsewhere in Europe, but abounds on the
opposite coast of America, where it is indigenous, and from whence the seeds | sporules [alternate
wording] have undoubtedly been borne across the Atlantic by the wind to the French coast. The

[103] It is self evident that the nearer to the infected body, the more concentrated the effluvia.

It may be safely inferred however from the great number of instances in which this form of fever occurs in single cases without spreading to attendants on the sick, that the sphere of activity of the virus is not nearly so wide as in the case of the eruptive fevers; and, as will hereafter appear, of the other form of fever which falls within the objects of this inquiry.

Reference to the great variety of conditions on which concentration of contagious effluvia depends will serve to explain many seeming anomalies in the propagation of this, as of [104] all forms of contagious fever.

The circumstances immediately relating to the virus of fever, that most favour diffusion of the disease, may therefore be reduced to these.

Plentiful production of the virus (as by malignant cases of fever or by the crowding of many in one place) in localities whose atmosphere is close and confined; — neglect by a large portion of the community of the common practices of cleanliness, and of every means for the removal or extinction of contagious effluvia.

To what appalling extent these circumstances are realised in the dwellings of the poor in large towns, we may gain some idea from the following graphic description from Willan's Reports.

During the mild open weather in January [1800], and at the beginning of February the Fever was again rapidly diffused to a very great extent, and with an aggravated train [105] of symptoms. Among the poor the mortality from this cause was very considerable, notwithstanding the attentive administration of proper articles of diet, and of suitable remedies, with plenty of wine. The good effects of these applications are often superseded by the miserable accomodations of the poor, with respect to bedding, and by a total neglect of ventilation in their narrow, crowded dwellings. It will scarcely appear credible, though it is precisely true, that persons of the lowest class do not put on clean sheets three times a year; that even where no sheets are used they never wash or scour their blankets and coverlets, nor renew them till they are no longer tenable: that curtains, if unfortunately there should be any, are

---

granules which propagate this plant are of almost microscopic minuteness. † The histories of the appearance of plants, even of large size, in localities in the neighbourhood of which they were previously unknown are full of curious analogy to the question of the spontaneous origin of fevers. (See Dr. Prichard's Physical History of Man. Vol. i.)

[James Cowles Prichard, *Researches into the Physical History of Man* (London, 1813).]

† Quote from Liebig — [illegible] — Fisk on salt forms

never cleaned, but suffered to continue in the same state till they
[106] drop to pieces: lastly that from three to eight individuals of different ages, often sleep in the same bed; there being, in general, but
one room and one bed for each family. To the above circumstances
may be added that the room occupied is either a deep cellar almost
inaccessible to light and admitting of no change of air; or a garret,
with a low roof and [small] windows, the passage to which is close,
kept dark in order to lessen the window tax, and filled not only with
bad air, but with putrid, excremental or other abominable effluvia
from a vault at the bottom of the stair-case. Washing of linen or
some other disagreeable business is carried on, while infants are kept
[sic, left] dozing; and children more advanced kept at play whole
days on the tainted bed: some unsavoury victuals are from time to
time cooked: in many instances, idleness, in others the cumbrous
furniture or utensils of— [107] trade with which the apartments are
clogged, prevent the salutary operation of the broom and white-
washing brush and favour the accumulation of a heterogeneous
fermenting filth. From all these causes combined there is necessarily
produced a combination of fetor to describe which would be as vain
an attempt, as for those to conceive who have been always
accustomed to neat and comfortable dwellings. page 254.[80]

I can state of my own knowledge, that this is still a faithful description of the dwellings and habits of the poor in London.[81]

The following account by Dr. J. Clark of the houses of the poor in
low parts of Newcastle is its counterpart.[82]

One poor family in these places seldom occupies more than one
room, and the [108] number in one family upon an average may be
computed at five. Their apartments in general have seldom more
than one window each, the sash of which is either entirely fixed or is
so constructed as only to open at a small part. One bedstead, a chair

80. [Robert Willan, *Reports on the Diseases in London Particularly During the Years 1796, 97, 98, 99,
and 1800* (London, 1801), pp. 254–56; [1800] added by Budd. Budd's emphasis — not in Willan.]
   81. (29) See Reports on the prevalence of certain physical causes of fever in the Metropolis by
Drs. Arnott, Kay, & Smith. (4th & 5 vol: of Poor Law Commissioners Reports.)
   82. † In reporting to government in 1837 on the causes of the existing prevalence of fever in
Ireland the physicians of the Fever Hospital on Cork Street thus express themselves —

   These do not differ in any respect so far as is known to them, from the causes of former
   epidemics already fully discussed & set forth in various reports presented to the Committee & to
   the public. The physicians have scarcely ever observed those circumstances which favour the
   progress of epidemic disease more strikingly exhibited than at present. They have frequently
   seen from 10 to 20 individuals crowded together in a single apartment of small dimensions, ill-
   ventilated, filthy and offensive in the highest degree, the inmates in want of the necessaries of
   life, often without bed covering or even sufficient personal clothing.
                                        p. 17 Alison in the Poor in Scotland

[Alison, *Management of the Poor.*]

and a stool are not infrequently the whole stock of furniture. The bedclothes are in general, scanty, tattered and dirty; and it is a rare thing to observe any change of bed-linen. Amongst the most indigent the bed clothes are never scoured, or the sheets washed; and an equal inattention to cleanliness is observed in their body linen: their rooms are seldom if ever whitewashed: the floors are dirty and the stairs and passages to them are filthy, dark and unventilated; the windows being for the most part blocked up.[83] (Page 2.3. Papers on Contagion).[84]

[109] It is easy to see with what powerful and certain effect the propagation of fever must be promoted by this lamentable realisation of the conditions most qualified to ensure the effect of contagious effluvia. But the evil is increased tenfold, especially as regards diffusion, when, as in lodging houses, the same conditions being present, a numerous succession of strangers is brought within their influence.

In the Report of a Committee of Inquiry "into the causes which produce, preserve, and propagate infectious fevers in Newcastle and Gateshead," the subject is adverted to in the following words.

The committee must observe before they leave this painful part of the subject, that there are lodgings [sic, lodging houses] the Longstairs, in Sandgate, Pandon, Pipewell-gate, in the High-street at Gateshead, and some of which there are often [110] at one time, from twelve to fourteen lodgers, two and sometimes three persons occupying the same bed. When a fever is produced in such houses, or when it is introduced, it rarely happens that any of the inmates [sic, inhabitants] escape [the] infection. And if a lodger die, or remove, he is succeeded by another who is put into the same bed, without any previous purification. It will be needless to mention the consequences, and to observe that those lodging houses more powerfully preserve and spread contagion, than perhaps the aggregate of all the other habitations of the poor.[85]

The above may be taken as a pretty faithful description of lodging houses in the low and dirty parts of large towns. It is to houses exactly answering this description that common sailors chiefly resort while in

83. (30) See also Dr. Currie on the dwellings of the Poor in Liverpool.† (Currie on Fever p. 347)

[James Currie, *Medical Reports on the Effects of Water, Cold and Warm, as a Remedy in Fever and Febrile Diseases*, 2 vols. (Liverpool and London, 1797-1804).]

† In Liverpool the poor mostly live in cellars.

84. [Clark, *Collection of Papers*, p. 6 – although the report may have been published separately, there are some variations in wording.]

85. [Ibid., pp. 8-9.]

port [111] in London and other large seaports. In these lodgings great numbers are attacked with fever; others having taken the infection fall ill in distant ports and there becoming new centres of contagion,[86] the diffusion of the disease is thereby immeasurably extended.

It is especially in severe winters when our rivers are for a season blocked with ice and the shipping detained in port, that seamen frequenting the class of lodgings described, are attacked with fever in vast numbers. This was particularly the case in London in the severe winter of 1838–39, when the Sea-men's Hospital was crowded with fever patients, for the most part, from lodgings in the low and filthy districts [112] adjoining the river. The magnitude of the evil thus arising, arrested the attention of the Committee of Management of that excellent Institution, and is earnestly adverted to in their Report of the following year, with a view to induce sailors to avail themselves more generally of the asylum which is offered them in the Sailors Home.[87]

Another circumstance connected with the necessities of the poor of large towns, and instrumental in the propagation of fever, requires notice here.

When a poor family has been further impoverished by visitation with fever, articles of clothes or linen, especially such as belonged to those who have died of the disease are either sold or pawned — Those who afterwards become possessed of these tainted articles receive unsuspectingly the [113] infection of fever.[88]

As evidence of the reality of this manner of propagation Dr. J. Clark

---

86. (31) I speak here advisedly and with sanction of numerous authentic facts which have come within my own knowledge.

87. * Recommendations more general

88. (32) All this is admirably delineated in the following passage from the Newcastle Report already quoted —

> In a neighbourhood, where a fever subsists, some person belonging perhaps to the family of a labourer or mechanic, from motives of humanity visits and assists the sick. In consequence of this infection is caught. The husband, after the disease is introduced, is often infected from attending his wife; and if the family have but one apartment, few escape the contagion. Poverty now presses hard on such a family; and if they have any stock of clothes or linen, they are gradually sold or pawned for their immediate support; and the unfortunate family, though in comfortable circumstances previous to the attack of this calamity, is soon reduced to a level with those originally in great indigence.
>
> But the evil does not terminate here; the clothes and linen sold or pawned, especially of those who die, are impregnated with contagion, as well as the room; and servants who visit their friends or acquaintances during the fever, and more particularly those who buy articles of linen or apparel from pawnbrokers, introduce the infection, without suspicion, into the families of the affluent. Such unsuspected modes of introducing contagion can seldom be traced; but that they frequently operate powerfully cannot be doubted.

[Clark, *Collection of Papers*, pp. 9–10.]

relates that the most malignant cases of fever he ever attended in Newcastle, were in the families of three pawn-brokers.

[114] In the cottages of the poor in the country there are also circumstances of great influence in promoting the propagation of fever. These circumstances, though less in degree, are the same in kind, as the more important of those just noticed.

In my own neighbourhood, most of the common labourers have but one bedroom: or if two, but one is generally occupied by the family. This room is low; without a fireplace and with one small window, either permanently closed, or opening by a very small lattice. There are generally three beds in the room. From scanty stock of bedding, not less than from want of clean habits [115] in the cottagers, the bedlinen is allowed to become very dirty before washed. Where sheets are used, (which is uncommon) they are washed but seldom; blankets and coverlets still more rarely; and I constantly have occasion to remark that after a contagious disease has run through a family of this class, no especial means are taken to purify the beds on which the sick have lain.

Thus close air and neglect of cleanliness are found in these cottages, ready to give effect to contagious effluvia. In some parts of the Kingdom, especially in Ireland, matters are still worse.

Also when typhoid fever occurs in the cottage of a common laborer, it generally attacks more than one of the family and often all who are susceptible of it — and if the neighbourhood be thickly inhabited and intercourse active, the disease may spread widely over the country.

[116] It appears from these details that conditions having immediate reference to the virus of fever: — increasing the concentration and activity of that virus and multiplying its forms of application, lay open to us when regarded in all their consequences, effects of wide and powerful influence in the propagation of this disease.

The wide spreading and fatal effects of the evil disclosed in that part of these details which refers to lodging houses in towns, urgently call for some remedy, and with stronger claim to attention, since the removal or mitigation of this evil does not seem beyond the scope and purpose of a well administered police.

[89] When we contemplate the frightful picture displayed in some of the foregoing descriptions, deep must be our regret that the dwellings

---

89. † [Opposite p. 116 the following note begins]

The Commissioners have seen frequent occasion to regret that the abodes of the labouring classes, & more particularly those in which the greatest proportn. of cases of destitution arise, are rarely visited, & in many districts are entirely [opposite p. 117] unseen and unknown by their

and habits of the poor are so ill-calculated for the casualties of contagious disease, and proportionately [117] earnest our wish that active benevolence, and capital may be more effectively directed to the improvement of those dwellings, and education more expressly applied to the reformation of those habits.

In accordance with the division I have adopted, I now pass to the consideration of conditions relating to the persons exposed to the action of the virus of fever, and which affect their liability to take the disease.

Discussing these conditions in order of importance, I begin with the protection against future attacks acquired to the system by one attack of this disease.

M. Chomel states that of 130 patients in typhoid fever, admitted into the Hôtel Dieu, there was not[90] [118] one who had ever had it before, and he adds that since this disease had been an object of special research in Paris, no authentic instance of its happening twice to the same person has been recorded. (Leçons Cliniques sur la Fièvre Typhoide. p:309.)[91]

M. Louis has lately informed me that although he has for a great number of years made diligent inquiry in regard to this point, he has not yet met with a single instance of the kind.[92] The great experience of this distinguished physician and unexampled accuracy of his method of inquiry give great weight to his statements. My own experience is precisely to the same effect. I have however been informed by friends of one or two authentic cases in which the disease happened twice to the same person.[93] On the whole I am inclined to believe that the protection

---

superiors in station. The facts set forth in the medical reports, to which the commissioners refer, were received with surprise by persons who were not aware of the condition to which their own labourers were living or of the neglected and dangerous conditions of their own immediate neighbourhood.

P.L. Commissioners to the Board of
Guardians of the Poor

[Great Britain, Poor Law Commission, "Sanitary inquiry."]

90. †[A note marked "p. 117, "Dr. Graves Medical Gazette vol XIX" was written on reverse. Robert Graves, "Clinical Lectures Delivered at the Meath Hospital," *London Med. Gaz.*, 1836, *19*, 570–71.]

["]It may originate spontaneously or from contagion — From what I have seen of it I have no doubt of its double origin. I am also inclined to think that it never affects the same individual more than once, & that when a man has had the true maculated fever, he never gets it again. In this point as well as in the eruption, it bears [close] analogy to the exanthemata.["]

91. [Chomel, *Clinique médicale.*]

92. [This passage suggests private correspondence or a visit to Paris, but neither can be substantiated.]

93. *I have an instance in my own house TJ [Thomas Jeffreys]

acquired by one attack of this fever, is [119] nearly if not quite as great as in the case of Scarlatina and measles.

The opinion generally entertained by the profession in this country is a considerable modification of that here expressed; for although it is believed by all qualified to judge, that one attack of fever confers some measure of protection for the future, that protection is thought to be much less than in the case of the exanthemata. But the credit this opinion has received, being, as will be shown in the next chapter, a necessary consequence of the general practice of considering in common the two forms of fever, which I have thought needful to separate, gives no motive for rejection of the opinion here adopted in accordance with the testimony of the French physicians.

The protection against this fever temporarily afforded to the system by the presence of some other [120] malady may be considered in this place.

M. Louis has made the important remark that typhoid fever is very rarely seen to complicate other diseases: — a truth which every practitioner may verify by reference to his own experience. It seems a fair and probable inference from the participation of various maladies in this common effect that febrile movement is the condition which confers this protection. However that may be, the reality of it is certain, and serves to explain the rareness with which fever is communicated from one person to another in general hospitals.

The influence of age is the next topic of inquiry.

The following table contains the experience of MM. Chomel and Louis in regard to the [121] age of 156 persons affected with this form of fever.

From the age of	15 to 20	there were	45
....	20 to 25	....	59
....	25 to 30	....	24
....	30 to 35 }	....	22
....	35 to 40 }		
....	40 to 52	....	6
			156

There was one only above 50.

In order to appreciate these numbers as indicating the degree of liability to fever in these several periods of life it is necessary to bear in mind that at each succeeding period the numbers of persons in existence diminishes and at some periods rapidly, while the number of those protected by a former attack of fever on the other hand increases. If the liability at each period were the same, the numbers attacked with fever, would represent the proportion of persons in existence at such periods minus [122] those protected by a former attack, and would give therefore a series of rapid decrement. But the second figure in the series exhibits an increase upon the first, indicating, a vast increase in liability from the age of 20. After 25 the figures decrease at each period more rapidly than can be accounted for as a joint effect of decrease in the number of persons in existence and increase of those enjoying protection and express therefore a real and progressive diminution of liablity as age advances. This diminution, very considerable from 25 to 30, increases very rapidly after 40, and would seem from these tables to amount to complete exemption before 55. The number of cases they contain is not sufficient however to establish absolute propositions with precise limitations.[94]

[123] M. Louis has lately informed me as the result of his accumulated experience that he has never seen typhoid fever after the age of 50. The only instance of this which I have seen was lately in a person 60 years old; but it is stated that M. Andral has seen it once in a person beyond 70.

The hospital experience of MM. Chomel and Louis does not extend to persons below 15: such being excluded from the hospitals in which these physicians practise.

The following statement of my late experience, in regard to this period of life may have some interest although not including a great number of facts. It refers to the ages of 32 persons who were attacked with fever in the epidemic of which I gave some account in the first part of this chapter.

---

94. (33) A valuable Report lately published by Dr. Jackson of Boston, United States, is I believe, rich in accurate statistics regarding the influence of age. I much regret that I have been unable to obtain it in time to avail myself of them.

[James Jackson, *Report Founded on the Cases of Typhoid Fever or Common Continued Fever of New England*, etc. (Boston, 1838). There is an additional note inserted opposite p. 122:]

† Porter des habits imprégnés de matière contagieuse, coucher dans des lits ou sur de la paille également infectés, c'est assez pour que dans l'espace [d'une ou] de quelques heures d'une chaleur uniforme, la contagion se développe chez des personnes saines, et surtout chez celles qui se seraient endormies.

p. 130

En considérant l'âge, nour voyons que les jeunes gens ou les personnes d'un âge moyen sont les plus disposés à la contagion du typhus. Il peut remarquer cependant que les petits enfants et les nourrissons qui contractent avec tant de facilité prêsque toutes les contagions, sont rarement atteints de typhus, lors même que leurs mères ou leurs gardes qui éprouvent cette maladie et qui viennent de l'essuyer depuis peu, sont en communication constante avec eux.

p. 141

[Hildenbrand, *Du typhus*, pp. 130, 141.]

Of these 32 persons fourteen were between [124] the ages of 10 and 20 — and of these fourteen 12 were fourteen years old and upwards — 5 between 20 and 30 — four between 40 and 60 — and nine below 10 years of age. The respective ages of the 4 persons beyond 40 were as follows,

42,
45,
50,
60.

Of those below ten there were 3 of 9 — two of 7 — two of 6 — one of 4 and one of two and a half years old.

These cases would seem to invert the inference drawn from the former tables in regard to the relative liability of the two periods following 15 years of age, but they are still more open than the others to the objection of being insufficient in number to establish general propositions. The decrease in the number of persons below [125] ten years of age, may however be safely taken as expressing a rapid diminution of liability from that period to infancy. I can state with certainty as the gross result of my experience and of that of many friends on whom reliance can be placed, that this form of fever is comparatively extremely rare below ten years of age. M. Chomel also states that although his hospital experience does not inform him on this point he has no hesitation in affirming that the number of persons attacked with typhoid fever progressively diminishes from five to ten years and that children under ten are very rarely affected with it.

When the vastly greater number of persons in existence below that age is considered, the great diminution of liability is plainly seen. [126] I believe it may be safely inferred from the foregoing statements that the liability to become affected with fever is greatest between the ages of 15 and 30; that it diminishes rapidly on both sides of this period and especially on that towards infancy: — that beyond the age of 55 this diminution amounts to all but complete exemption.

As regards the liability of Childhood this differs widely from a statement published by Dr. A. S. Thomson in the Edinburgh Medical and Surgical Journal. 1838.[95]

It there appears as the result of a calculation that persons below 10 years of age are much more liable to fever than persons of any age above

95. [A. S. Thomson, "A Statistical Inquiry on Fever, etc." *Edin. Med. Surg. J.*, 1838, *50*, 87–118.]

it.[96] [127] This result is another of the consequences, of which I have to notice so many, arising from the practice of considering in common the two forms of fever: a practice which introduces error into almost every part of the inquiry thus prosecuted. Nearly all statistical accounts of fever [128] that have been attempted on a large scale in this country are chargeable with this pervading error.

From these and previous considerations it follows that the conditions most favourable to the spread of fever are the occurrence of cases in localities where ventilation is difficult, and where those exposed to effluvia from the sick are persons in early manhood.

These conditions are often realised in the Navy, especially on the breaking out of War, and in the fatal epidemics of fever that ravaged the Channel Fleet we had sad experience of their consequences. Yet these dreadful consequences might have been easily averted by the appointment of an hospital ship, to which the first cases might have been removed. The frequent [129] neglect of that precaution, in our war with the French, after experience had proved the need of it, and assured its efficacy serves to show what great sacrifice of health and life is sometimes needed to force upon public authority, the practical application of established and important truths.

By the wise precautions now observed in manning the Navy, fever seldom finds its way into our Fleets, and the services of an hospital ship are in great measure superseded by War Steamers which are ready to receive the first cases of contagious disease and to transport them to hospitals on shore.

This is however a time of peace, but should war again break out and the exigenc[i]es of the Service not allow of the precautions now observed in manning the Navy,[97] [130] fever, if epidemic on shore, might again appear in our Fleets and the present establishment of Steamers be insuf-

---

96. (34) This result is also obtained by a process to which there are fundamental objections. The number of cases upon which it is founded is not the result of actual observation, but a calculated number | thus obtained [added]. Having ascertained the proportion of deaths for a limited number of cases in an Hospital, in Glasgow, Dr. A. S. Thomson uses this proportion to calculate from the number of deaths from fever recorded in the bills of mortality, the whole amount of cases of fever occurring in Glasgow in a twelve month! This method appears to me to imply a total misapprehension of the use and purpose of Statistics. The great purpose of Statistics is by drawing results from large numbers of observed facts to diminish the chances of error that may and often must affect the results of a more limited number. But by the method here followed the errors that may thus arise are multiplied instead of corrected.

97. † [There is inserted a note marked "p. 129" which repeats what was said earlier]

From several of these cases, especially those of the sawyers, it would appear that the latent period of this fever is usually ten days at least. There is no doubt however that {the} its duration {of this period} is subject to great variation: — variation {contagion on} contingent on a number

ficient to prevent its spread. Should such circumstances be realised it is to be hoped we shall profit by the experience of the late war.

If by the observance of wise precautions, fever seldom or never finds its way into the Navy, by the culpable neglect of all precautions it is ever breaking out in those ships that transport our emigrant poor to distant Colonies. In these ships, as in the Navy, the persons congregated are for the most part in the prime of life and therefore the most disposed to receive the infection of fever: and by criminal evasion of the Law for the base purpose of gain | cupidity [alternate wording], they are [131] closely crowded in low and contracted cabins. The dreadful consequences are now well known: the fatal spread of fever among the poor emigrants, the introduction of it into our colonies, and the necessity of maintaining expensive quarantine establishments to mitigate this evil, have been ably set forth, and successfully forced upon the attention of the legislature, by persons high in authority.[98]

Persons attacked with typhoid fever being for the most part of the working class, — in the prime of life and therefore heads of families, prevalence of this disease has an especial effect on the poor rates and increases pauperism more than any other.

[132] Sex.

Materials are wanting by which to determine with certainty whether or not liability to fever is affected by sex. The collection of such materials is open to numerous and fruitful sources of error not hitherto guarded against by any one who has investigated the subject. There is no presumption however that liability to fever is materially affected by sex.

Various degree[s] of liability of different persons, and of the same person at different times.

Analogy teaches us that different persons vary greatly in their susceptibility of contagious diseases. In the case of Smallpox these varia-

---

of conditions, of which the principal one seems to be the amount of virus received by the system — All this is well exemplified for the other form of fever by the series of cases given in an admirable paper on the subject by Dr. Marsh, (in the 4th volume of the Dublin Hospital Reports) and in many of which it was quite evident that the disease followed immediately on reception of the virus. — There is further analogy {for this} in the case of smallpox and also, though more remote in the case of marsh fevers. I have now before me a case of smallpox caught by single exposure in which the latent period was extended to 5 weeks — The great variation of the latent period of marsh fevers is well known.

98. (35) See Lord Durham's Report on Canada. — also — The Emigration Reports.
[Great Britain, "Report of the Earl of Durham [John George Lambton] on the Affairs of British North America," PP, 1839, XVII, 1 ff, also published separately (London, 1839). The report was

tions are most distinct to observation. Some persons seem to enjoy complete immunity from that disease; [133] immunity testified by repeated failure of inoculation and by exemption from the disease under frequent and unguarded exposure to its effluvia.[99] Others on the contrary are prone to receive it in confluent form under slight exposure, and even to take it a second time. This unusual susceptibility is often found in many of the same family, and evinces as Dr. Holland has justly remarked a disposition that may be transmitted hereditarily,[100] however the intimate nature of the conditions on which that disposition depends may elude our search.

[134] Although more difficult of proof, there is little doubt of similar variation in liability to typhoid fever. Many persons take this disease on slight exposure, while others remain exempt from it during long continued and unguarded exposure to the effluvia of fever patients. Variations of similar kind and independent of that which I have shown to be the effect of age is observed in regard to the same individual at different times. Here again the conditions on which this variation depends for the most part elude observation.[101] It has been alleged that debauch and exhaustion of all kinds increase liability to this disease, and curious facts have been adduced in illustration of this statement.[102] There is also analogy to support this in the fact stated by P[arent] Duchatelet, that

---

prepared by Charles Buller. The "Emigrant Reports" are Great Britain, "Report from the Select Committee Appointed to Inquire into the Expediency of Encouraging Emigration from the United Kingdoms," PP, 1826, IV, 1 ff, and 1826-27, V, 112-222, 223-882.]

99. (36) In an Epidemic of smallpox at Norwich, Mr. Cross, who has given us an excellent history of the Epidemic, found that of 215 persons liable to smallpox, there were 15 (or 1 in 14 1/3) who escaped the disease although under continued and most intimate exposure. [John G. Crosse, A History of the Variolous Epidemic Which Occurred in Norwich, in the Year 1819, etc. (London, 1820).]

100. (37) I have seen an instance in which 3 brothers took smallpox a second time and 2 of them died of it.

101. † [Opposite p. 134 the following notes are inserted:]

Dans l'été de 1809, pendant que je rédigeais cet ouvrage, se montrait déjà au commencement de la guerre une contagion générale analogue, qui menaçait de devenir dangereuse pour l'avenir. Le germe s'en développa en partie par l'encombrement des logemens des militaires, en partie par la mauvaise situation des camps, et enfin par les hôpitaux même, d'où elle se répandit ensuite par les évacuations et les différentes marches des convalescens, de manière à produire les plus grands ravages. On pouvait suivre et décrire la direction qu'avait prise cette maladie, par la route qu'avaient tenu ceux qui en étaient infectés. p. 26

Ils sont encore présens à la mémoire les malheurs qu'ont produits les guerres dans ces dernières années par la mortalité à la suite des contagions. Après les campagnes de 1793-94, les maladies contagieuses, désolèrent l'Allemagne [(1)] et elles se renouvelèrent dans les années 1796-97. Après la campagne de 1805, une contagion meurtrière parcourut toute la Galicie, la Moravie, la Bohême, la Hongrie, l'Autriche, et pénétra dans l'Allemagne et dan la Russie. p. 25.

[Hildenbrand, Du typhus.]

102. (38) See Lind on Contagion & Fevers

persons under these circumstances are more liable to the [135] deleterious effects of the noxious air of Sewers. (Page. 138. op:cit:)

The influence of want of the necessaries of life,[103] and of public
calamity, in increasing liability to the disease is perhaps more certainly
assured by the fact, that most of the great epidemics of fever whose
history has been accurately written, have occurred in times of scarcity,
or other public calamity. I may refer to the epidemic of 1817 in
Ireland — of 1826 in Scotland — to that of Genoa described by Rasori —
and to those referred to by Hildenbrandt [sic], as remarkable
Examples.[104]

103. * This circumstance too lightly noticed

104. † (Inserted facing pp. 135-38 perhaps as a result of the adjudicators' marginal comment
relating to this paragraph]

[Facing p. 135] When I say that I consider the repeated occurrence of extensive epidemic
fever as a clear indication of great previous suffering among the poor I am perfectly aware that
the assertion may be open to some objection. We all know that contagious fever may exist, and
spread to a certain extent where there is no destitution; and we know also that destitution may
exist (although I believe never for a length of time and in a large town) without fever showing
itself. I believe also that fever extends much more rapidly, or possesses a stronger contagious
property in some seasons than in others, in all ranks of the community. It is not asserted that
destitution is a cause adequate to the <u>production</u> of fever (although in some circumstances I
believe it may become such); nor that it is the sole cause of its extension. What we are sure of
it, that it is a cause of the <u>rapid diffusion</u> of contagious fever, & one of such peculiar power &
efficacy that its existence may always be presumed, when we see fever prevailing in a large
community to an unusual extent. The manner [facing p. 136] in which deficient nourishment,
want of employment & privations of every kind; and the consequent mental depression favour
the diffusion of fever may be matter of dispute; but that they have that effect to a much greater
degree than any cause external to the human body itself is a fact confirmed by the experience of
all physicians who have seen much of the disease. Alison on Management of the Poor in
Scotland. pp. 10-11.

That it is always in persons suffering, or who have lately suffered, similar privations &
sufferings & the mental {despondency} depression & despondency which naturally attend them
that continued fever becomes extensively prevalent is fully established by the history of all
considerable epidemics — The elaborate work of Drs. Barker & Cheyne shews that this has been
{the case with al} strictly true of all the great epidemics which have appeared in Ireland since
1700, each of them lasting fully two years; viz. in 1708, 1720 & 1731. in 1740-41 (after the
great frost [facing p. 137] of 1740), in 1800-1. after the rebellion, the transference of the seat of
Government to London & the scarcity of 1799 & 1800. and again in 1817 after the transition
from the state of war to that of peace & the scarcity of 1816-17. That work contains reports
from the most eminent physicians in all parts of Ireland on that great epidemic, all agreeing in
the statement that the poor were the greatest sufferers, & the fever seemed to rage among them
'in {proportion} a degree proportionate to the privations they had endured.' In Ireland accordingly, at least during the present century, as the general condition of the poor has been
decidedly worse than either in England or Scotland, so contagious fever has never ceased to be
more generally prevalent. The same observation applies to the epidemic fever in London after
the scarcity of 1800 — to the great epidemic continental fever of 1813-14 which followed the track
of the French Army retreating from Russia but never made much progress in the victorious
allied army, to the [facing p. 138] epidemic fever in Italy consequent on the scarce year of
1816 — to the epidemic which affected the British Army in Holland after the disastrous retreat
from Flanders in 1794, — in Portugal after that from Burgos in 1812, — & to that which nearly
decimated the British Legion in Vittoria in 1836. — Ibid. p. 11-12

(The effect of the same causes illustrated by the Scotch epidemics)

The connexion of fever with destitution appears from the observation which I have myself
made many hundreds of times in the Old Town of Edinburgh that it is among those of the poor

Influence of Season.

Much difference of opinion has arisen respecting the influence of season on the prevalence of fever, and both the amount [136] and kind of such influence has been very variously estimated. Autumn has been generally considered the most favourable to the spread of this disease. Dr. Currie states however as the result of his experience that fever is most prevalent in March and least so in August, but he remarks afterwards in reference to the fever in Liverpool that "on the whole the prevalence of fever is greater and the influence of season less than might have been expected." (p. 355, Currie on Fever.) [105]

But it is especially in regard to the influence of low temperature and frost that we find the widest difference of opinion expressed by authorities on the subject; some asserting the great power of cold and frost to check the spread of fever, others, to promote it. [106]

This great and manifold difference of [137] opinion has arisen in part from a general disposition to overrate the influence of season and in part, and especially in regard to the point last mentioned, — from the practice of studying this influence on the spread of fever without reference to the different forms of the disease.

It is evident from considerations developed in the foregoing discussion of the various circumstances which affect the spread of fever, that the influence of season must be subordinate to many of these, and may often be rendered insignificant by their predominant effect. Such is the case not only with typhoid fever but also with all contagious diseases as appears from the occurrence of extensive epidemics of these diseases at various seasons of the year. [107] [138] By observation of these epidemics physicians are however led to the adoption of corresponding | [corre]lative [alternative wording] opinions regarding the influence of Season, and thus have arisen the differences already noticed.

The influence of season whatever it may be, can only be determined

---

who suffer the greatest privations, — whose employment is precarious, often suspended, or little profitable, — and among disabled men, low women, widows and orphans, especially among the poor Irish, or other strangers of this descript[ion], that fever most frequently appears, and always spreads most rapidly and {fatally} extensively. Ib. p. 14–15.

[Alison, *Management of the Poor.*]
105. [Currie, *Medical Reports.*]
106. (39) See Blane, Batemen, Tweedie, and others.
107. (40) The following is but one of countless illustrations —
Pendant que Sydenham trouvait que la petite vérole était plus violente et plus maligne dans la canicule, on observait en France une épidémie de [la] petite vérole qui enlevout beaucoup plus d'individus dans l'hiver que dans l'été. (Lamotte, Traité complet de Chirurgie, tom:III)
[Guillaume Mauquest de La Motte, *Traité complet de chirurgie*, 4 vols. (Paris, 1732).]

by extensive averages of observation | including a considerable lapse of time [added], referring separately to each form of fever. Such as we are in possession of indicate the autumnal months, from August to December, as those most favourable to the spread of the form of fever considered here. My own Experience, as far as it goes, exemplifies [139] this, both in regard to the occurrence of sporadic cases, and of Epidemics.

All the epidemics of this disease that have come within my immediate observation, have happened in these months.

I have already alluded to the wide difference of opinion which exists regarding the influence of low temperature. Facts will be stated in the course of this Essay giving strong presumption that the spread of the other form of fever is promoted by cold, so that the difference of opinion alluded to would be satisfactorily explained were it shown that the observations of those, who consider cold unfavorable to the spread of fever, referred to the form of fever under present consideration.

The influence of high temperature is I believe better ascertained. In the [140] numerous Squadrons fitted out for the West Indies during our war with the French, and in which fever prevailed so much, the decline of the disease on reaching warm latitudes was too marked and too constant to be the Effect of chance. The testimony of Sir G. Blane and of Dr. Trotter to this Effect is uniform and decisive.[108]

The following passage expresses Sir G. Blane's experience in regard to this — "The ships which bring this fever from Europe in general get rid of it soon after arriving in a warm climate, and nothing but the highest degree of neglect can continue or revive it." p. 249.[109]

The mention of spontaneous diarrhea as a frequent symptom leaves little [141] doubt that these observations refer, for the most part at least, to the form of fever here considered. In the instance of one Squadron that doubt is entirely removed by the statement that "erosions and even holes" were found in the intestines of one man who died of this fever. (See p:137-345 Diseases of Seamen). At page 147 of the same work is a statement which implies that Sir G. Blane was familiar with this kind of lesion as an effect of this disease.

---

108. (41) See Blane on diseases of Seamen pp: 62, 242, 341, and Dr. Trotter, Medic: Nautic: Vol: I. pp. 190, 195, 203.
[Gilbert Blane, *Observations on the Diseases of Seamen,* 3d ed. (London, 1799); and Trotter, *Medicina nautica.*]
   109. [Blane, *Observations,* p. 250.]
   (42) See Hunter on Fever. Medical Transactions Vol:III
[John Hunter, "Observations on Jail or Hospital Fever," *Med. Trans. Roy. Coll. Phys.,* 1785, *3,* 345-67.]

Briefly stated, our knowledge of the influence of weather and season amounts to this — The power of great heat to check the propagation of this fever is well ascertained and considerable: and it seems probable that extreme cold has a power of the same kind, but less in degree.

Autumn is the season most favorable [142] to the spread of this disease.

It is plain that the agency of weather is not simple but may depend on the various conditions of atmosphere relating to humidity, density, currents, temperatures and electric state, and that these conditions may operate in affecting the liability of the human body to the influence of the agent producing fever, or in modifying the intrinsic activity and manner of diffusion of that agent; or which is probable, in both ways.

We are not in possession of Elements whereby to appreciate the separate effects of these several modes of action. It is likely however that temperature is principally concerned in the influence of hot weather, and that it takes effect chiefly on the agent producing the disease seems probable from what we have cause to presume of the [143] nature of that agent.

Impure Air.

Although it cannot be admitted that typhoid fever may be caused by miasmata generated in the decomposition of organic matters yet it is possible that breathing air contaminated with these miasmata, may render the human body more liable to the action of the specific cause of this disease.

The specific cause of Cholera certainly has greater effect in places where the air is thus corrupted.

It is also probable that where persons ill of fever breathe air of this quality, their disease affects a more malignant type, and I have already shown good reason to believe that a greater amount of virus is generated in malignant cases of fever than in mild ones.

[144] In both these ways impure air may possibly promote the spread of fever. Notwithstanding all however that has been so confidently asserted of its influence, satisfactory proof of that influence is, it must be acknowledged, entirely wanting. Considerations already developed in this chapter in connexion with other circumstances which promote the spread of fever, plainly show that the effects attributed to air corrupted with putrid effluvia, may be for the most part, if not all, explained upon other grounds.

I have now passed in review all the circumstances that can be distinctly recognised as affecting the propagation of this form of fever. They have been found in great number [145] and various importance: some of powerful influence, and each susceptible of great variety in degree and effect. Looking to the endless variety of Effect that must result from the various combination of so many Elements, each fluctuating in importance, we are at no loss to account for all the seeming anomalies which the history of this disease exhibits, and for every degree of prevalence in which it is observed: from the occurrence of isolated cases, seeming without power to multiply by contagion, to the spread of epidemics through large masses of population.

These seeming anomalies, and various degrees of prevalence are a necessary effect of the complexity of the elements concerned.

For want of due regard to this complexity and clear perception of its necessary consequence, Medical [146] Inquirers have been led, by the diverse character of the facts which the history of this disease exhibits, to conclusions which that diversity by no means involves. One of the most remarkable of these, and the only one which remains for me to notice, is embodied in the current opinion, that this disease may in some cases be contagious and in others not, by virtue of intrinsic change in its nature or evolution, effected by various and trivial circumstances. This opinion is negatived by a just appreciation of the special nature of this property of multiplying by Contagion, — is discountenanced by analogy, and the facts on which it rests may be otherwise and satisfactorily explained by reference to the considerations developed above.

This is indeed a case in which analogy is decisive.

[147] Facts exactly similar to those on which the opinion in question is founded might be alleged to show that smallpox is in some cases contagious and in others not, by virtue of intrinsic change in its nature; — a conclusion the absurdity of which is here made plain by the tangible form in which the virus is generated.

I have already stated with as much precision as the subject admits, the conditions necessary for the communication of fever from one person to another.

Some of the conditions passed in review, as capable of affecting the spread of this disease, claim more particular notice in their application to the circumstances of Epidemics.

The protection acquired to the system by one attack of fever, has important [148] bearing on this part of the subject.

When great numbers of a given population have been attacked in the course of an epidemic, and the sickness afterwards declines, — partly on account of immunity enjoyed by some, — of the insufficient exposure of others, and partly on account of various other circumstances less distinct to observation, it is plain that the population from which fever has thus retired, will by virtue of the protection conferred on those who have been infected, be less liable to a similar irruption, until a sufficient lapse of time shall have restored the former proportion of persons liable to the disease. The Exact period of the next outbreak will, in some measure be a matter of casualty, and contingent on a great variety of circumstances, such, for Example, as the character of [149] the neighbourhood in which the early cases may occur, just as the extent of a conflagration depends on the nature of the materials along which the first Spark may fall.

CHAPTER 3RD.

Inquiry into the causes and mode of propagation of that
form of typhoid fever in which there is no specific lesion
of the intestinal follicles and which is often attended
with a measles-like eruption.

As in the special works on fever that have been written by physicians
of this country, the specific identity of this form of fever with that last
treated of has rarely or never been questioned, but these two forms have
been considered in common; our standard works contain very few
documents that can be safely used [151] as having exclusive reference to
either form. It was on this account that I thought right to avail myself in
the last chapter of facts observed in places abroad, where this source of
confusion does not exist, deeming myself justified in that course by the
certain identity of the disease to which those facts relate with that which
was the object of research.

Evidence relating to these forms separately would, on account of
their general resemblance in symptoms, be very difficult of attainment in
this country, were it not that in some large towns epidemics of one form
sometimes prevail to the almost total exclusion of the other, as was mentioned in the first chapter of this Essay.

Some excellent observers have favored us with narratives of
epidemics of this kind, and these narratives contain [152] almost the only
precise information touching on this form of fever, that we are yet in
possession of.

Unfortunately these are few, and the facts they set forth not sufficient in number to form a secure basis for general propositions.

During two years I have had much opportunity of observing this
form of fever and the statement of my own experience together with that
recorded in the narratives alluded to, must in the absence of more ample
evidence, form the ground work of the following considerations.

In the Introductory Chapter I have already referred to Dr. Alison's
narrative of the epidemic of this form of fever that prevailed in Edin-

burgh in the year 1826-27.[1] It will be remembered that in the fatal cases examined by [153] him there was complete absence of specific lesion of the intestines.

In correspondence with this, constipation was the most common condition of the bowels during life. A majority of the cases also exhibited a rash "closely resembling what is seen in the contagious exanthemata particularly the measles" — The statements in this narrative may therefore be safely adopted as referring to the form of the fever to be considered in this chapter.

In November 1826 it was determined on account of the great increase of fever in Edinburgh and Leith to fit up Queensberry House for the reception of fever patients, and to appropriate an increased number of beds to the same purpose in the Royal Infirmary.

The history of these two [154] establishments during the Epidemic that filled their wards abounds in proof of the contagious nature of this form of fever.

At Queensberry House the resident physician, two clinical clerks, the apothecary, several servants, and all the nurses but two; — in all above 40 persons attendant on the sick, were attacked with fever.

Now this must have been either the work of contagion or of some malaria pervading the house and independent of the sick therein. If a malaria it was a very virulent one and as Dr. Alison well remarks it is reasonable to expect that some record of similar visitations would be found in the former history of the building. But in the lapse of a century, during which Queensberry [155] House was occupied, first by the noble family of that name, then by several families, and afterwards as a soldiers' barrack, it had never been visited with an epidemic of fever.

In the Royal Infirmary six of the clerks employed in the clinical wards, four of those in the ordinary wards, and 25 nurses or servants were attacked with fever. All these persons but four were by reason of their duties in close and immediate intercourse with the fever patients. Of these four two had been employed in the laundry where the linen from the fever wards was washed. One was a porter who had communication with the fever patients, at their entrance and dismissal; the other a nurse in the habit of frequently visiting the fever wards. [156] That this extension of the disease to attendants on the fever patients, was not the effect of malaria but of contagion, was made plain by the exemption of those inmates of the Infirmary that had no intercourse with the

---

1. [William P. Alison, "Observations on the Epidemic Fever Now Prevalent among the Lower Orders in Edinburgh," *Edin. Med. Surg. J.*, 1827, *28*, 233-63.]

fever patients. Of the inhabitants of the ground floor none but those mentioned as having washed the linen from the fever wards and the barber who shaved the heads of the fever patients were attacked with this disease: nor any one of the nurses, whose duties confined them to the Medical or Surgical wards where no fever patients were admitted.

Dr. Alison also relates two remarkable instances, in which this fever was evidently imported into previously healthy districts of the town by persons who had come from distant quarters of it and were just recovered [157] from the disease. In one of these instances the repeated migrations of a family could be traced at every change by a trail of infection.

To this conclusive evidence Dr. Alison adds cumulative proof furnished by facts of negative order. I shall here quote his words:

> It is quite clear, that if the succession of cases in limited districts depended on a malaria in each, these successions should be equally apt to take place when the first patients were removed as when they remained at home during their illness. But while it is, as I have already said, exceedingly rare to see a case of fever run its course in any of the crowded districts, without other cases speedily following in the immediate vicinity, nothing is more common than to [158] see single cases not followed by any others, when they are removed to the hospital within a few days from their commencement. What was stated as the result of my [own] experience in the New Town Dispensary during the former epidemic is strictly applicable to all that I have seen in the present. We should have little difficulty in pointing out above a hundred houses where a single case of fever has occurred, where the patient has been speedily removed and the place cleaned, and where there has been no recurrence. But we should hardly find five houses in all the closes of the Old Town in which a patient in fever has lain during the whole or even during half of his disease and in which other cases of the disorder [sic, disease] have not speedily shown themselves. (See pp:242. 28th Vol: Edinburgh Med: and Surg: Journal.) [2]

[159] Not only do these facts, taken together, contain sure evidence of the propagation of this form of fever by contagion but as Dr. Alison well remarks it is difficult to understand what better evidence can possibly be expected.

I need not relate in detail facts to the same effect that have fallen under my own observation or that have been recorded by others.[3]

---

2. [Ibid., pp. 242–43; "[own]" added by Budd]

3. (1) See a paper by Dr. West on typhus exanthemata in Edinburgh Med: & Surg: Journal for April 1838. [Charles West's paper, "Some Account of the Typhus Exanthematicus in St. Bartholomew's Hospital, London, in 1837–38," appeared in the July 1838 issue of the *Edinburgh*

Those already brought forward are authentic and conclusive: addition to their number is therefore needless. It will be sufficient to state that the evidence they contain is supported by the concurrent testimony of all who have had much [160] opportunity of observing this fever.

Also in Cities in which it prevails its contagious nature is regarded, by all qualified to judge, as an established truth.[4] I shall therefore recognise it as much, and proceed at once as in the former chapter to consider the consequences that may be deduced therefrom. Many of the reflections made in that chapter apply with equal fitness here and need not therefore be repeated.

It would be easy to prove by appropriate facts, that the air is the medium through which the virus of this fever is most commonly communicated from one person to [161] another and that concentration is the condition which most certainly ensures the specific effect of this virus. It would be no less easy to show that the virus may be harboured in tissues, or other articles of furniture, in effective quantity and form. These data involve the same train of deductions that was followed in the former Chapter, and which led us to recognise in the dwellings and habits of the poor, the conditions most apt to promote the operation of contagious principles.

In regard to the period at which in this form of fever emission of contagious effluvia begins and ceases, or is most abundant: as also the length of time these effluvia may remain active after separation from the infected body, we must confess the same ignorance as was expressed [162] in regard to these several points in connexion with the other form of fever. Hildenbrandt [sic] was of opinion that this disease acquired the faculty of spreading by contagion on the first appearance of the rash, and not before. He does not state the grounds of his opinion which were probably speculative only.

There is the same presumption for this as for the other form of fever, of a more abundant emission of contagious effluvia in malignant than in mild cases.

In the former Chapter I pointed out the impracticability of deter-

---

Medical and Surgical Journal (50, 118–45).] Barker & Cheyne's history of the Epidemic of 1817. A paper by Dr. Marsh in The Dublin Hosp. Reports Vol: IV: [H. Marsh, "Observations on the Origin and Latent Period of Fever," *Dublin Hosp. Rep.,* 1827, *4,* 454–536.]

4. (2) The evidence afforded by the Epidemic of 1837–38 in London and Edinburgh was of a kind to convince the most inveterate unbelievers of contagion. We may repeat with Hildenbrandt [*sic*] the following apt remark. "On connaît chaque jour davantage la nature contagieuse du typhus, et le sceptique ne fait, à cet égard, que témoigner le défaut d'observation." (p: 275 French Translation)

mining, in terms of measurement, the sphere of activity of contagious effluvia diffused in the air, and the prejudice to inquiry that has resulted from [163] attempts to do so.

The range of activity of the contagious effluvia of different diseases may however be compared with sufficient precision, and such comparison will be found a source of instruction. I have no doubt, from my own observation, that the form of fever under present consideration, is more highly contagious than that form which is attended with special alteration of the intestinal follicles. This statement will, I am confident, receive the sanction of those who have seen most of these two diseases; as indeed I have assured myself, by consulting many eminent physicians, attached to hospitals in London, Dublin and Edinburgh.

In consequence of this more active propagation there are fewer sporadic or single cases of this than of the other [164] form of fever. Indeed it may be safely affirmed that this form of fever never happens sporadically, in the strict sense of that term, and that single cases of it are nearly, if not quite, as rare as of scarlatina and measles.

When the considerations on spontaneous origin, that were developed at so much length in the former chapter, are brought to mind, it will plainly appear that the circumstances attending the propagation of this form of fever, do not give presumption even, that this form has any origin other than contagion.

The difference in degree of contagious activity here set forth, as existing between the two forms of fever, will account for the great diversity of opinion prevalent as to the origin and [165] propagation of fever generally. In Paris and some other places, where that form attended with intestinal affection is observed alone, and where there are no fever hospitals, the contagious nature of fever is very generally discredited; — in our own Country the opinions of medical men vary according as one form of fever falls under their observation to the more or less perfect exclusion of the other.

Those who see fever in the country, where that form with intestinal affection most generally prevails, have for the most part, doubts of its contagious nature: whereas those, who in some cities, have had their attention absorbed by epidemics of the other form, believe in contagion as the sole origin: — others again whose experience has been of mixed kind, [166] while they recognise the contagious nature of fever, assert that it also originates spontaneously.

These various opinions have already been discussed at sufficient length in these pages. I shall not therefore indulge in further remarks upon them in this place, but pass on to the consideration of conditions having immediate relation to the persons exposed to the virus of this fever, and affecting their liability to the disease.

In this I shall follow the arrangement adopted in the foregoing chapter, and begin by discussing the degree of immunity for the future enjoyed by a person who has once had the disease.

There is some diversity of opinion in regard to this point, among those best qualified to judge, but I cannot doubt, from my own knowledge [167] and from numerous statements made to me by persons who have seen much of this fever, that instances of recurrence in the same individual are much more common than in the case of the other form of fever.[5]

This also accounts very satisfactorily for the difference of the opinions in regard to this point held by the French physicians and our own.

Instances are indeed alleged of recurrence of the form of fever under present consideration, three and even four times to the same individual, and several such have been related to me with every semblance of authenticity by persons who had themselves been the subjects of such repeated attacks.[6] There is no doubt however that an attack of this disease greatly [168] diminishes the liability of the subject to be again affected. I am inclined to believe that the amount of protection thus acquired is considerable, but materially less than in the case of Scarlatina and measles, and of the other form of fever.

Influence of age.

The following table contains a statement of the ages of 342 patients admitted without selection into Queensberry House during the epidemic of fever referred to in the first part of this chapter.

Under 15	83
From 15 to 30	149
... 30 to 50	93
Above ... 50	17
	342

[169] From this table it would appear that liability to this form of fever is much greater between 15 and 30 than at any other period of life. How

---

5. [Epidemics of relapsing fever were still described as typhus in 1839.]

6. [Robert Christison, one of Budd's teachers at the University of Edinburgh, often made this claim in arguing against the exanthemata analogy.]

much less it is below that period is plainly seen when we consider the great increase in the number of persons living as we descend the scale of age. But the number of persons below 15 given in this table is undoubtedly much too small to express the real proportion of persons attacked with this fever below that age, for parents are extremely reluctant to send children of tender age to hospitals. The real proportion can be determined only by accurate returns from Dispensaries.

It may be stated however as certain that liability to this disease diminishes rapidly below the age of 15.

In early life then, liability as affected by age varies [170] according to the same law nearly for both forms of fever, but in later periods there is a notable difference.

It will be remembered that of 156 cases of fever observed by MM: Louis and Chomel there was but one in a person above 50, and the age of that one was 52, whereas among the 342 (little more than the double of 156) whose ages are given by Dr. Alison there were 17 above 50. These numbers are undoubtedly too small to warrant any general inference, but I place great reliance on their indications because my own experience fully bears them out. In a very extensive epidemic of this form of fever which I once witnessed, cases were common in persons above 50 and not rare in persons of 60 and upwards.

Influence of Sex

Of 677 per- [171] sons attacked with this form of fever and admitted without selection into Queensberry House there were,

Females	397
Males	280
	677.

These numbers do not indicate with certainty that the liability of females is absolutely greater than that of males, for women are by their habits and by their acts in the capacity of nurses much more exposed than men to effluvia from the sick.

Season and Weather.

Still quoting from Dr. Alison's narrative I subjoin the number of fever patients admitted during each month from November 1826 to July

1827 inclusive, into Queensberry House and the Edinburgh Royal Infirmary.

As not one fever patient was refused [172] admittance during that period these numbers express pretty accurately the general variation in the prevalence of fever according to each month during that epidemic. The whole number of cases were 1570 and they were distributed as follows,

November	146
December	201
January	211
February	242
March	236
April	176
May	128
June	90
July	130
	1570

It will be seen that the number of cases increased rapidly from November to December, and was greatest in the depth of winter, diminishing again with the advance of Spring.

[173] I believe this to be the expression of a general fact. Dr. Alison states that in all former epidemics which he had witnessed the number of sick increased greatly on the approach of winter. The same has been again observed in Edinburgh in an epidemic which began in 1835 and continued to prevail for three winters, gradually declining as Spring advanced, and, except in 1836 almost disappearing in Summer.

Speaking of the number of admissions into the Royal Infirmary during that epidemic Dr. Henderson says,

Cold weather had commonly the effect of increasing the number of admissions which declined again when the temperature was moderate. These fluctuations were noticed not merely on a general and large scale as on comparing the effects of summer and winter, but even in [second page numbered 173] the latter season occasional changes of weather though not persisting above eight or ten days had the effect I have mentioned.[7]

7. (3) See Edin. Medic: and Surgic: Journal: Oct: 1839. How strongly opposed are these facts to the hypotheses that fever is produced by effluvia from the decomposition of animal and vegetable matters.

[Henderson and Reid, "Report on the Epidemic Fever of Edinburgh," *Edin. Med. Surg. J.*, 1839, *52*, 429-62.]

In the epidemic of fever which occurred in London in 1837–38 and reached its height in the depth of the severe winter of that year, the great mass of the cases was of that form of fever considered in this place.[8] There is little doubt therefore that winter, and cold weather generally, are extremely favourable to the spread of this fever; a fact which as I have already said, [174] furnished another point of difference in the history of the two forms.

It is clear that winter may promote the spread of this form of fever in various ways. It is probable that no inconsiderable part of its effect is due to the circumstance that at that season a great number of artisans are out of employ, and passing a greater portion of their time in their own dwellings, are thereby more exposed to the effluvia of such inmates as may happen to be ill of fever.

The operation of those effluvia is also rendered more certain by the close state in which these dwellings are then kept in order to shut out the cold.

The increase of want and general distress which is the necessary consequence of so many being out of employment, must also contribute [175] to the same effect. But it is probable that winter has some more direct effect, for it has been shown that the spread of the other form of fever is rather checked than promoted during that season. I have already mentioned a circumstance favourable to the spread of fever during winter, peculiar to those seaports in which navigation is liable to be obstructed by ice.

From observations made in a former chapter it seems probable that hot weather may check the spread of this disease, by dissipating contagious effluvia and thereby rendering them less active.

I have now passed in review all the circumstances which it has seemed to me necessary to consider as [176] affecting the origin and propagation of this fever.

The conclusion established in the first part of this chapter, that contagion is the sole origin of this form of fever, allowing me to apply to this form many of the considerations relating to that origin that were developed in regard to the other, has enabled me to dispense with a great number of details, and to treat briefly of these circumstances. And to this I have been in some measure compelled by the scantiness of materials

8. (4) Sir Gilbert Blane notices an epidemic which seems to have been of the same kind as occurring in the unusually severe winter of 1735.

which I have had such continual occasion to regret. Fortunately this scantiness concerns, chiefly, points of minor importance.

In this review I have been led to the recognition of some material points of difference in the conditions [177] that affect the spread of this and of the other form of fever: — recognition more important, however, as tending to clear away sources of confusion that vitiate current opinions, than as having practical bearing on the general objects of this inquiry.

In the conditions of greatest practical bearing, those, namely, relating to contagion, and to the period of life most liable to fever, there has been found almost perfect agreement.

CHAPTER 4TH

Recapitulation.

The two principal forms of typhoid fever whose causes and mode of propagation have been considered in the foregoing chapters, include all the varieties of the common continued fevers of this country that I am acquainted with, unless it be certain febriculae or ephemeral fevers, that are induced by common causes of sickness; — have no faculty of propagating by contagion, — are of short duration, — not epidemic, — and altogether of trivial importance.

[179] Those chapters contain therefore such answer as my humble abilities have enabled me to give to the question proposed in the first page of this Essay.

It now only remains for me to collect together and express in general terms, the elements of this answer that are dispersed over the preceding pages, and there set forth in detail.

Led at the outset to recognise two principal forms of fever, differing in many important characteristics, if not in species, it was thought necessary to treat separately of the causes and mode of propagation of these two forms.

That form attended with specific alteration of the intestinal follicles was treated of in the first place. [180] Numerous and authentic facts were brought forward proving incontrovertibly a power in that form to propagate by contagion. From this was deduced the important and leading truth, that the proximate cause of that form of fever is, in all cases, a material and specific agent or virus.

A series of facts was also brought forward, giving evidence of the frequent occurrence of cases not traceable to an immediate prototype, and under every semblance of spontaneous origin; furnishing presumption therefore that the specific cause of the fever, although in many cases the product of the peculiar vital processes constituting the disease, — as was shown by the faculty of contagion, — might also be the offspring of some other and alien process.

On further consideration of these facts; — borrowing for their interpretation the [181] help of analogy; — recognising in the provisions found
in society for secret dissemination of contagious principles, admissible
grounds for their explanation; — and lastly confronting the presumption
first derived from them with various objections, — that presumption was
found to lose much of its original force and to fall very far short of proof
of the production of the specific cause of this fever in any source other
than the infected body.

Still less was it considered proved that this specific cause is really the
offspring of certain sources, — such as the decomposition of organic matters for example, — in which it is commonly supposed to be bred.

Those sources, to which the production of this specific cause has
been imputed with greatest plausi- [182] bility and highest sanction,
were, next, expressly considered; and after deliberate and I trust, fair
examination, it was thought necessary to reject the grounds of that
imputation.

These several parts of the inquiry received further illustration in the
course of the Chapter in which they were introduced.

The chief points that were established, therefore, in regard to the
form of fever attended with specific lesion of the intestines, were, that
this form has power to propagate by contagion, and is caused by a
Specific Virus.

That if this Virus have any other source than the infected body, that
source has not yet been discovered, [183] and the infected body is the
only one that can be distinctly recognised.

In regard to the other form of fever, which was also shown to propagate by contagion, and to be caused by a specific virus, no presumption
arose of the origin of that virus in any source other than the human body
infected with it.

From these considerations it appeared, that, as far as the specific
causes are concerned, the only conditions that, in our present state of
knowledge, can be distinctly recognised as affecting the origin or spread
of these fevers, are such as affect the production and effect of contagious
effluvia.

In the study of these conditions I was led to remark in the dwellings
and habits of the poor, of large towns especially, [184] an appalling
realisation of all the circumstances most apt to multiply the outbreaks
and promote the spread of contagious diseases. It was further shown how
the effect of these circumstances is multiplied and immeasureably

extended by their presence in lodging houses, especially where these, as in seaports, are the resort of common sailors.

Of the conditions that affect the liability of persons subjected to the action of the specific causes of these fevers, to become affected thereby, the most influential were found to be age, and the occurrence of a former attack.

The prime of life, was shown to be the period most liable to the attack of both [185] forms of fever. The influence of this was exemplified by reference to the annals of the Navy, and to the frightful spread of fever that often takes place in Emigrant Ships, in which great numbers of persons in the prime of life are crowded together. The wide-spreading influence of the evil thus incurred was explicitly noticed.

The occurrence of one attack of either form of fever was shown to confer some measure of protection against a recurrence of the same form, and that protection was considered to be much the greater in the case of the fever that is attended with intestinal affection.

The especial relation of this acquired protection, to the periodical [186] occurrence of epidemics was fully developed.

Other conditions of less influence and less distinct to observation were also recognised as affecting the liability of persons to the attack of these fevers.

The principal of these were want of the necessaries of life, as exemplified by the remarkable spread of fever in times of general scarcity, — debauch and exhaustion of other kinds; and, but of contrary effect, the presence of some other malady.

In discussing the influence of climate and weather I was led to observe that this influence is subordinate to other circumstances of greater moment, and may be lost in their predominant effect. [187] Such influence of climate and weather as may be observed, was shown to differ somewhat in effect on the spread of the different forms of fever.

A hot climate and hot weather generally, were shown to be unfavourable to the spread of either form; for the form attended with intestinal lesion this was shown by reference to the experience of the Navy; for the other form, by the evidence of various epidemics observed in this country.

In the influence of winter and cold weather a notable difference was remarked: the winter season and severe weather being highly favourable to the spread of the form last mentioned and unfavourable to the spread of the other form, which, for the most part, prevails in the autumnal months and seems generally to [188] decline on the setting in of severe weather.

Such is a summary of the opinions advanced and statements made, in the foregoing pages. Many of them are I well know in direct opposition to opinions that have long been generally received, that have repeatedly been favoured, in various countries, with learned and distinguished sanction, that have enlisted zeal in their promulgation, and hot passions in their defence. I am not so sanguine as to hope that anything here advanced, will obtain preference over opinions, thus sanctioned by time and learning, and cherished by warm predilections. The varied and perplexing character of the facts which it is the object to explain, may, however, well give scope to variety of opinion, and tends greatly to diminish the weight of authority in favour of any given doctrine. [189] On this account I have been less diffident than I might otherwise have been in the assertion of opinions; however adverse to the doctrines that enjoy general as well as distinguished favour.

In conclusion I may be allowed to state that I approached the consideration of this subject with a deep sense of its great difficulties, with consciousness of the peculiar nature of the evidence here needed for the attainment of truth, and of the utter hopelessness of any progress towards that attainment unless the mind of the Inquirer were beforehand purged from all bias and prejudice. I trust that in the conduct of this Inquiry, however imperfect my success, I have continued to act under the influence of these sentiments.

THE END.

December 27. 1839.

AFTERWORD:

THE STUDY OF CONTINUED FEVER IN VICTORIAN BRITAIN

The questions concerning fever in the 1840s were of two sorts: first, the degree of difference between the different forms of continued fever and the evidence to be used in establishing the answer, and second, the source(s) and mode(s) of propagation. The second question was by far the most important to Victorian physicians and public health activists. The first, the degree of difference, emerged as important only when it impacted on the second, or in the case of a few practitioners, generally Paris-trained, interested in the science of pathology as an end in itself. This priority is seen in Davidson's winning essay, but also in Budd's conclusion — he had demonstrated "two principal forms of fever, differing in many important characters, *if not in species.*"[1] Budd certainly believed in an essential difference, but it was based not solely or primarily on the pathology but on the facts that both of the principal forms were spread by contagion and the causes were obviously different since only one of the two appeared in a given epidemic experience. Whether it was called a species-level difference was not overly important in an era when the definition of species was somewhat fluid. What was important was that one fever did not give rise to the other form under any circumstances, so, in the sense that species propagate only their own kind, the two fevers were separate species.

In country districts such as North Tawton, the fever epidemic of 1839 was clear and the results unambiguous. Nevertheless, most medical theorists did not practice in villages but in cities, where the industrial revolution produced large migrations of people, crowding, slums, and unsanitary working places. William Budd clearly recognized in his essay that he could not study the form of fever without intestinal lesions in North Tawton. Furthermore the village did not offer sufficient scope for the aspiring young physician, and he began to look for other opportunities.

In 1840 Budd earned an appointment at the *Dreadnought* but caught a fever and during the autumn became very ill. He was forced to resign his

post and return to North Tawton to recover his health. During his convalescence, he began to expand and revise his 1839 prize essay, a process
on which he was still at work twenty-three months later, after he had
moved to Bristol to establish an independent medical practice.[2]

At Bristol, William Budd's practice developed slowly, and he had
time to devote to researches on various aspects of medical science, but,
probably because he lacked further firsthand knowledge of the forms of
fever, he did relatively little with his essay. In 1843 he read it, or parts of
it, to the Bristol Medico-chirurgical Society. In 1842 he was appointed
one of the physicians to St. Peter's Hospital — the facility maintained by
the Board of Guardians — and in 1845 was elected a lecturer in medicine
in the Bristol Medical College, a non-degree-granting faculty. In 1847
Budd was elected to the staff of the Bristol Royal Infirmary, a more
prestigious hospital and position than the poor law one at St. Peter's. He
was reported so pleased by his appointment to the infirmary's staff and
the opportunities for clinical research that it provided that "he could
hardly restrain himself from setting off to run, in his anxiety to see how
his cases were getting on."[3] But Bristol, once the second city in the
kingdom, had been passed by; the industrial revolution had come first
and foremost to the north. Bristol had its poor, even a few Irish immigrants, but conditions were not severe enough for endemic typhus to be
a major problem. Budd occasionally saw the disease in epidemics at St.
Peter's Hospital, but he was unable to gain real familiarity with it. He
became even more familiar with typhoid fever, which was endemic in
Bristol, and it is for his contributions to the understanding of the
epidemiology of typhoid fever that he is best remembered.

As Budd clearly recognized in his 1839 essay, any real knowledge of
etiology and epidemiology of fever was dependent on accurate diagnosis
and the concept of specificity. He had attempted to establish the
nonidentity of continued fevers on the basis of his knowledge of typhoid
and his limited experience with typhus in Edinburgh, London, and
Dublin but recognized that the final proof was left "for those who have
opportunities of observation in places where both forms are
common. . . ." The essential question was whether "one communicates
the other," but that could be resolved only in London or in the industrial
cities of the north.[4]

Glasgow was one such city, and there Robert Perry's ideas continued
to exert an influence. In 1840 Andrew Anderson published his thesis,
Observations on Typhus, in which Perry's explanation of the medical events
was reproduced with evidence from the local hospitals. Dr. Anderson

argued that there were two distinct diseases: typhus fever, a general disease the pathology of which was unknown, but which was a specific and contagious illness; and dothienenteritis, a local inflammation of the small bowel. The two could and frequently were combined in the same patients to produce a typhuslike fever with a localized intestinal complication accompanied by abdominal symptoms, but the resulting combined disease did not differ from typhus "as typhus is from smallpox, for example; that is each being a *fever,* properly so called . . . but . . . like typhus and pneumonia, perfectly heterogeneous. . . ."[5] Unless the dothienenteritis were equally contagious with typhus and the two spread in the same way, the experience of the country practitioner, like that of William Budd in the North Tawton epidemic, made Anderson's theory impossible, but in a city where both diseases were generally endemic to some extent and both occasionally epidemic, it was quite possible to believe in the theory of Drs. Perry and Anderson.

The distinction between typhus fever and dothienenteritis, once drawn, as it had been in Glasgow, did provide incentive for further study. The result of such study and broader experience may be seen in the 1840 paper of Alexander P. Stewart on the distinction between typhus and typhoid fever. This essay, read at Paris in April 1840 before the Parisian Medical Society, was undertaken to describe leading features of the difference between typhoid fever of Paris and the typhus normally seen in Scotland. Stewart, a student of Louis, believed they were "totally different diseases," basing his argument in part on the pathological and clinical differences described by Gerhard, Stillé, and Shattuck, but more importantly on the differences in the origin and causes of the maladies.

Stewart, on the origin of typhus, followed the ideas of theorists of the Fever Hospital Movement and the sanitary reformers, ascribing typhus to the effluvia of animal matter given off in large quantities by people in crowded circumstances. This he found to be totally different from the Paris experience, where fever was not obviously related to crowding or slums but struck those new to the city. Further, he argued that typhus in Britain was generally believed to be contagious but that the fever of Paris was not thought to be so.[6] Stewart raised questions but was not emphatic or forceful in his resolution of the problem. His evidence was interpretative, and he failed to convince his contemporaries in large measure because of his selective use of the evidence. While typhus was considered to be frequently contagious, it was also considered to be generated de novo under the proper conditions. Furthermore, the typhoid fever of the

French, while less contagious or less frequently so, could be spread from
the sick to the healthy in exactly the same way as British typhus; the
experiences of Pierre Bretonneau at Tours and James Jackson at Boston
were cited by one reviewer to prove Stewart wrong.[7]

The difference of diseases based on the difference of some symptoms
and the anatomic pathology was not particularly well received either. In
the pathological study of the distinction, Stewart with Budd and a third
Louis student, H. C. Barlow, suffered from a serious misunderstanding
of the nature of pathological anatomy as practiced by Pierre Louis.[8]
Louis's term "anatomical character" was read by most British physicians
of the 1830s and 1840s as "cause." In one review of Louis's second edition, the idea that Louis believed typhoid fever to be the result of a local
inflammation of the intestine was described as "almost invariably" held
by English physicians. The majority of practitioners saw the fever
debates in terms of the essentialist vs localist controversy of the previous
generation; Louis was characterized with Broussais and Clutterbuck as a
localist.[9] As long as pathological anatomy was perceived in this limited
way, the evidences of postmortem analysis were not convincing. What
was important to most practitioners was therapy, and to many, therapy
meant relief of observed symptoms. In such circumstances, the symptomatic similarities were more important than the relatively minor
symptomatic differences. This was the view that caused William Cullen
to group all variants of typhus together in his eighteenth-century
nosography,[10] and in the practical considerations of Alexander Tweedie
and William Davidson it produced essentially the same result.

The practical emphasis was made plain in the early Victorian period
by the writers in the *Library of Practical Medicine* (Robert Christison) and
the *Cyclopedia of Practical Medicine* (Alexander Tweedie). In these very successful publications, fever was an essential disease that exhibited complications of the cerebral, thoracic, or abdominal organs. In France the
abdominal complications predominated, but in Great Britain the various
complications were all seen depending on the particular epidemic influ-
ences.[11] Even those with a better than average appreciation of the nature
and role of anatomic pathology were confused by the febrile experience
and feared the localist interpretation of Louis's research. Thomas
Hodgkin wrote:

> If we admit the facts which I believe Professor Louis to have drawn
> up with conscientious accuracy, I do not see how it is possible to
> evade the conclusions at which he has arrived. . . . It appears to me

to be altogether presumable that the inculcation of the doctrine, that
in fever the glands of Peyer at the termination of the ileum are
always in a state of inflammation; and that, on the other hand these
glands are never affected but in cases of fever, may lead many to
adopt the conclusion, that the inflammation of the aggregate glands
in question really constitute the essence of fever.[12]

This fear of the abuse of anatomic pathology in practice was very
real and justified by the experience of the 1830s, when leading British
physicians were attempting to institutionalize pathology in the changing
British medical curriculum. But the key problem always reverted to
causation, and, because pathological explanations were of secondary
importance, it was possible to compromise. This sort of compromise is
evident in a review published in 1841 on the question of the identity or
nonidentity of the continued fevers of France and England, in which the
reviewer concluded, "We believe, then, that the continued fevers of both
countries are the *same species* of disease; but they are *different varieties* of
that species."[13]

The reviewer went on to note that there were problems left to solve,
which were largely related to the cause and spread of the fever. Why
should the form with lesions be so universal in France but not in
England? How could the experiences of John Reid of Edinburgh, where
lesions were rare, and John Goodsir at Anstruther, thirty miles away,
where the lesions were universal, be explained or reconciled? Why did
the proportion of cases with intestinal lesions vary so widely from season
to season and epidemic to epidemic? These questions were resolved by
the absolute distinction, as species, between the forms of continued
fever, but the anomalies raised by such a solution were considered worse
by most practitioners. Such a solution raised diagnostic difficulties
without providing therapeutic guidance and upset the carefully balanced
etiological ideas that had grown out of the experience of fever epidemics
and the constant presence of endemic fevers in the poorer sections of
cities. As long as the decision was a matter of choosing which set of problems to leave for further study, most practitioners chose the epidemiological ones raised by the 1841 reviewer. The professional consensus is
perhaps best illustrated by William Farr, whose successful nosology
stressed the limitations of the anatomic definition of fever and favored
the physiological union of "all modified forms of fever."[14]

In 1843 the matter of choice was taken out of the hands of the
medical profession by the widespread recognition of an epidemic of fever
in Scotland that was unlike the continued fever generally called typhus.

The first cases probably occurred late in 1841 or early in 1842 on the east coast of Fife; in the summer of 1842 the disease was epidemic at Dundee. The first cases in Glasgow occurred in September 1842, and before the end of the year the epidemic was widespread there. In February 1843 it appeared in Edinburgh, and at about the same time in Aberdeen. The disease also occurred in smaller towns in Scotland and in some cities in England. There was a marked increase in admissions to the London Fever Hospital in 1843, and some attempt at retrospective diagnosis suggests the disease was the same as the Scottish epidemic but was not so recognized at the time.[15]

While many observers recognized that the 1843 epidemic was not the same disease that they customarily experienced, it was the work of the Edinburgh medical profession that had the most pronounced impact. The earliest notice of the significant differences between the usual fever and the epidemic was a short note by William P. Alison. Alison noticed that the cases of epidemic fever were of much shorter duration, generally lasting from five to seven days; did not have the typical eruption of typhus fever; and were frequently jaundiced and had a greater tendency to nausea. There was considerably less mortality than he expected, only one case in thirty terminating fatally, despite extremely high morbidity. Most peculiar of all, though, was the very pronounced tendency to relapse. After the disease "ended" in a sweating crisis five to seven days into the illness, the patient remained sore, and the disease returned, usually on the fourteenth day. There was also a pronounced tendency for pregnant patients to abort.[16]

Alison, by the mid-1840s committed to reform of the Scottish poor law and the relationship of poverty and disease, saw only that the epidemic of 1843 struck the poorest of the poor and thought that it had its origins in the habits and habitats of the poor. His views, formed in the epidemics of the post-Napoleonic era, which may have been primarily the same disease, had been voiced repeatedly in the late 1830s and 1840s as the sanitary reform movement developed in England, but they could not be maintained as the evidence accumulated that the disease was so unlike the usual typhus as to be considered a different species of disease.[17] The disease of 1843 went under a variety of names; initially it was described as a new fever and identified with Thomas Sydenham's *nova febris* of 1685; it was also called short fever, five-day fever, seven-day fever, bilious remittent fever, remitting icteric fever, mild yellow fever, and synocha; but it was known most frequently as the relapsing fever and was soon recognized as the same form of fever that had been epidemic in 1815–19, and that had led Dr. Benjamin Welsh to believe in the ability of bloodletting to cut short typhus.[18]

Because of the presumed newness of the fever and its striking differences from typhus, as well as its epidemic occurrence, the relapsing fever of 1843 attracted the attention of almost all the major medical practitioners of Edinburgh and many of those in other Scottish cities.[19] One of Dr. Alison's colleagues at the Royal Infirmary, David Craigie, published an account of his experience with the disease over the summer months in 1843. He drew four important distinctions between the relapsing fever and the usual typhus and synochus of Edinburgh. Relapsing fever had a strikingly different clinical course in that it was of shorter duration and the patient tended to relapse; it failed to show the red spots characteristic of typhus; it was not associated with delirium or hallucinations; and, while exhibiting extremely high morbidity, it had a very low mortality. Dr. Craigie outlined the typical clinical course of the disease, described its progress through the summer, and attempted to clarify some confusion concerning the diagnosis. Some of Edinburgh's physicians who had spent time in the West Indies had drawn attention to the similarities of the 1843 epidemic, with its tendency to nausea and jaundice, to the yellow fever of the tropics. Dr. Craigie was careful to show the variety of distinctions between the two, probably in an effort to forestall confusion and potential panic.[20]

Dr. Craigie considered the question of the mode of propagation of the disease and noted that many considered it contagious, but he thought that the conclusion was "rather a presumption than a well-found inference." Like Alison, Craigie drew attention to the fact that the disease struck most heavily in the "most densely inhabited" areas of Edinburgh, those "very favourable for the origin and propagation of a disease depending on atmospheric causes." Furthermore, it seemed to have occurred almost simultaneously in several Scottish cities. He did acknowledge that information received from Glasgow, where many of those nursing the sick had been taken ill, suggested that the disease might be contagious, but he thought that the proportion of such cases in Edinburgh was too small to draw any positive conclusions from them.[21]

By December 1843, when Professor William Henderson summarized the distinctive nature of the 1843 epidemic before the Medico-chirurgical Society of Edinburgh, the situation was clearer. Henderson explained the difficulties that had made the study of inquiries into fevers so slow and unsatisfactory. The first was that in all continued fevers there were certain common symptoms that led to their classification as fevers — symptoms much more striking in their singularity than any differences among them. The second great difficulty was that the fundamental pathology of fevers was completely unknown; all pathological theories put forward were inadequate to explain the phenomena. Finally, there had been relatively little effort to study carefully and scientifically the circumstances that produced fevers.[22]

The last difficulty was, for Henderson, the most important, and its resolution in terms of the relapsing fever epidemic of 1843 was the key to unlocking the mystery of continued fever in Britain. By December 1843 Henderson probably suspected that the first two difficulties, distinctions among symptoms and in pathological anatomy, had been established at least partially in the immediate past. Physicians had distinguished typhus from typhoid fever on both primarily symptomatic (Robert Perry of Glasgow) and primarily pathological grounds (H. C. Lombard, W. W. Gerhard, A. P. Stewart, etc.), but rarely on etiological grounds. Pierre Bretonneau had drawn such distinctions at Tours, and William Budd's experience at North Tawton was being discussed by the medical profession at London, but Henderson may have been unaware of both. Even if he knew of the work of Bretonneau or Budd, their ideas might not have meant as much to him as a situation where more than one form of continued fever was present, as at Edinburgh in 1843.

Henderson acknowledged that differentiation on a basis of cause alone was inadequate; many physicians believed that "the same disease may acknowledge in different persons several different causes, and the same cause may occasion very different diseases." Yet there were limits to such latitude — "certain diseases can be produced but by one cause, and certain causes can produce but one kind of disease" — and when that limit was attained, then causation provided grounds for distinction. In the case of continued fevers, Henderson argued that although nothing was known about the actual nature of the cause, it was admitted that continued fevers were caused "by some poison or other," even if the poison were held to be unspecific. If such a doctrine were carried to extremes, it became absurd. As examples, Henderson cited Marsh's claim that the contagion of smallpox could produce typhus and the contagion of typhus, intermittent fever, or the equally foolish belief of Dr. Thomas Southwood Smith, who argued that intermittents, remittents, typhus fevers, and plague originated from different intensities of the same poison.[23]

As a criterion Henderson advanced the following suggestion: "Suppose we should find two fevers, strikingly dissimilar in many important characters, prevailing at the same time in a community, and both of them undeniably infectious, if we find in the case of persons infected with either, the disease, of which kind so ever it may be, clearly traceable in each case to infection received from persons labouring under the same disease, like producing like, have we not just grounds for concluding that . . . they must be essentially different?"[24]

Henderson then recounted his experience with the epidemic of 1843 in an effort to establish that the usual typhus and the relapsing fever were distinct symptomatically and etiologically. First, he established the differential diagnosis, emphasizing the clear difference in symptoms — "the very first cases which fell under my notice I distinguished, at once, as widely different from every fever that I had formerly seen." To the distinctions already drawn by Alison and Craigie, Henderson added that in relapsing fever the pulse rate was much higher than was usual in typhus, and further that rapidity of pulse in typhus was indicative of a bad prognosis, while the relapsing fever was a mild disease.

Henderson was careful to establish that typhus occurred at the same time and in its characteristic form, noting that during the summer of 1843 he had taught students on the wards to distinguish the two diseases and that his definition of typhus conformed to that of other practitioners. The one recourse of the unitary fever theorist not easily and generally eliminated was the invocation of individual peculiarities, but Henderson was able to provide examples of people who had, within a relatively short space of time, suffered from both the relapsing fever and the typical Edinburgh typhus.[25]

Finally, Henderson described his efforts to trace individual cases, fully recognizing that he had not been able to follow every case to its source of infection and that he had obtained some apparently contradictory results. Nevertheless, he argued that if fevers were the same and had the same cause(s), "cases of typhus and of the epidemic fever should be found to spring up or to be mixed up together inextricably." But they did not. Henderson had been able to trace twenty-nine of thirty-nine cases of typhus he had seen since the epidemic of relapsing fever began in February; in only four cases were there any indications that the patient had been in contact with patients suffering from relapsing fever. In one instance, in which a patient had been sent from a lodging house where there were cases of relapsing fever, it was determined that the girl had been wandering from place to place and had probably not been in the infected house long enough to have caught the disease there. In the other three, Henderson found evidence of exposure also to typhus. In three of the remaining twenty-five cases, no source of exposure to either form of fever could be identified. In the remaining twenty-two, Henderson found "a succession of cases of typhus occurring in the same household, unmixed with the epidemic fever, and in some instances, of typhus communicated from one household to another surrounded with the epidemic fever."[26]

One of these series may be quoted in extenso to illustrate the type of evidence that Henderson believed was needed:

> A boy, Thomas Lynch, became affected with typhus fever, in a stair in Stevenlow's Close, on the 29th of July. He was attended by Mr. Lee, and the exanthematous eruption was ascertained to distinguish his disease. There had been nine cases of the epidemic fever in the stair previously, but none in the same house, which was occupied by eight individuals, two of whom were lodgers. On the 1st of August, James Lynch, also a boy, took the same disease. On the 26th of August, Daniel Brady, who was seen by Mr. Lee lying in the bed with the two boys when they were ill with the fever, became affected with the disease, and was subsequently under Dr. Alison's care in the Infirmary, where I had an opportunity of seeing him, and of ascertaining that he had typhus fever, with the usual eruption. On the 2d. of October, a sister of Brady, also a lodger with the Lynches, began to complain, and was afterwards admitted into the Infirmary under the care of Dr. Graham, who recognized her disease as typhus fever. No cases of the epidemic fever appeared among these people at this time, and when they were last visited in November, no other individual had become affected with the typhus, and the epidemic fever had not yet attacked them. Among the other families in the stair, however, the latter disease had spread extensively, but without any examples of typhus.[27]

Henderson had established his diagnosis and had it independently corroborated; he had further established the opportunity of contagion and had shown that each disease produced only cases of the same form. He acknowledged that in December 1843 his efforts might be "labouring to prove what none are now inclined to deny,"[28] but he was also establishing a model of what would be needed in the further study of continued fever in Britain. Henderson's remarks illustrate the true magnitude of the realization that continued fever in Edinburgh was not one disease that appeared in various forms, but at least two diseases. It was a realization shared by many Scottish practitioners in 1843, and the experience had a profound effect on fever research.

The man who took up Dr. Henderson's model and finally resolved the controversy over the identity or nonidentity of continued fevers was William Jenner, who was completing his M.D. degree requirements at University College, London when Henderson's paper appeared. Jenner had initially qualified as an apothecary, but in the early 1840s had returned to University College to qualify as a physician. [29]

When Jenner graduated in 1844, Thomas Watson's textbook of medicine, published in 1843 but written originally in 1836-37, contained the latest information on medicine and was rapidly becoming a standard authority. Watson, in company with most authorities in England, believed that while "fever shows itself under various forms . . . the effect upon the mind of all this subdivision is bad and hurtful. It encourages a disposition, already too prevalent, to prescribe for a disease according to its name. There is no line of genuine distinction between continued fevers that can be relied upon. They run insensibly into each other, even the most dissimilar; and are traceable often to the same contagion." [30]

Yet progress was being made. In 1843 William Budd read a paper on his North Tawton experience before the Bristol medical society. After 1845 Budd taught at Bristol that typhoid or intestinal fever was a specific contagious disease, and in later editions of his textbook Thomas Watson referred to Budd's ideas, albeit briefly. [31] In 1842 at Lowell, Massachusetts, Elisha Bartlett wrote a monograph on the differences between typhoid fever and typhus, which was reviewed in Britain, generally unfavorably, in the mid-1840s. [32] Finally, the mid-1840s were a period of intense discussion of sanitary reform as a result of Edwin Chadwick's 1842 report, but the discussion did not concern current research in pathology. Instead the question that preoccupied public health authorities was the nature of the spread of disease. The sanitarians remained largely unaware of changes in medical opinion that had occurred over the previous twenty years. The opinion accepted by most persons in the public health movement was that described as contingent contagionism. [33]

During the early years of his practice, Dr. William Jenner was called to see a young lady suffering from severe abdominal pain. He asked for a consultation "with one of the most able physicians of the day, a man of great experience." The diagnosis was acute idiopathic peritonitis and the case terminated fatally. At a postmortem the practitioners found "tolerably extensive ulceration of Peyer's patches, and enlargement of the mesenteric glands; in fact, the anatomical characters of typhoid fever."

Where lay the fault? Had the physicians been unable to diagnose the case properly because medical science was unable to provide the criteria, or were they "behind the age in the information" that they used? Jenner recalled that he determined to find out and began an extensive study of fever.

William Jenner found that there were two opinions in the literature — firstly, that all continued fever was identical as to species but variable according to various complications and circumstances, or secondly, that confounded within the designation *continued fevers* were two or more distinct diseases. The answer was not available in the literature, although there was a strong suggestion among all who had done extensive investigation that various fevers were distinct. Jenner applied to Dr. Alexander Tweedie for permission to observe the practice of the London Fever Hospital and to conduct postmortem research on fatal cases. Tweedie, who was as concerned as anyone to establish the facts relating to continued fever, gave Jenner every facility for four years, from 1846 to 1849.[34]

Late in 1849 William Jenner published his results, but while he had been working other investigators had also been active. Most promising were the researches of Dr. Charles Ritchie of Glasgow, who in 1846 coined the term *enteric fever*. Ritchie was a longtime practitioner in the Glasgow area, at first as an apprentice-trained general practitioner in rural areas and then as a fellow of the Faculty of Physicians and Surgeons. In 1837 he had been a member of the expanded committee of the Glasgow Medical Society that had reviewed the observation of Robert Perry on the distinction between typhus fever, an essential, systemic disease, and dothienenteritis, a local inflammatory disease of the small bowel.[35]

At the August 1846 meeting of the Medico-chirurgical Society of Glasgow, Charles Ritchie gave an extemporaneous address on fever. He believed that there were two basic forms or genera — simple continued fever and typhus. Simple continued fever was caused by environmental factors and, depending on the cause or causes, could affect different organs or one organ system more prominently than others. Such differences were not of the same generic level but could be considered as species of simple continued fever and called cephalic, bronchial, gastric, gastro-hepatic, and enteric. Such species were convertible one into another, but never into typhus. The subject was continued until the September meeting, when Ritchie read a prepared comparison of typhus and enteric fevers to illustrate his ideas.[36] Following the original work of

Dr. Perry, Ritchie outlined both the similarities and differences between the two fevers. The principal differences were that typhus was usually the result of contagion, whereas enteric fever was not. Typhus was believed to have a longer incubation period. The symptoms differed. Typhus was more a derangement of the nervous and sensory organs, while enteric fever was primarily an affliction of the intestinal tract. The postmortem appearances differed; both the lungs and the digestive system were more prone to changes in the enteric fever patients.[37] The paper, published in 1846, contained no explanations; it was simply the outline of similarities and differences prepared for the society meeting, although the final means of difference was the need for different therapies. Ritchie did not seem interested in justifying his exercise. His paper appears to have been without influence.[38]

In 1848 Edward Latham Ormerod published a monograph on the pathology and treatment of continued fever as it occurred at St. Bartholomew's Hospital, London, where he was demonstrator in morbid anatomy. Ormerod argued that it was true that the various local pathological changes made possible the differentiations of fever into subgroups, but it was important to recognize the similarities evident in virtually all cases. He acknowledged the existence of fever but went on to consider the local complications as the most important points in pathology and therapy because no natural pathological whole could be described for general fever. Ormerod's work follows Tweedie's organ classification in examining the attack of fever and its various secondary affections in order — brain, lungs, abdomen.[39]

In his 1849-50 work, William Jenner considered all aspects of continued fever. First, he confirmed the observations of Gerhard, Shattuck, Stewart, and Barlow on the symptomatic and pathological differentiation of typhoid and typhus fevers. He defined the question of identity or nonidentity of the various forms of fever by analogy with the exanthemata — smallpox, scarlet fever, and measles. A distinct disease might vary widely in the symptoms presented in a particular case; a mild sore throat and *scarlatina anginosa* were both scarlet fever. Yet scarlet fever and smallpox, which everyone acknowledged to be distinct diseases, were sometimes confused. Jenner observed, "So like too is the rash, which often precedes by a day the eruption of the pustules in smallpox, to the rash of scarlet fever, that those conversant with the two diseases may be led to form an erroneous diagnosis." How then was a decision to be made? Jenner believed that five criteria might be used — in the majority of cases the symptoms differed; the eruptions, when present, were never identical; the pustule or anatomical character of smallpox was *never* seen in scarlet fever; while both were contagious, in no combination of circumstances could a case of one disease produce a case of the other; and finally the epidemic constitution that favored epidemics of one had no effect on the other disease.[40]

In his effort to establish the identity or nonidentity, Jenner took the anatomical character of typhoid fever as defined by Louis as a given. He then examined the records of all fatal cases that had been autopsied to determine whether a difference in symptoms accompanied a difference in postmortem findings. Of his total experience from 1846 through 1849, Jenner had only sixty-six cases with complete clinical records and autopsy results; these divided into twenty-three cases of typhoid fever, that is, fever with Peyer's patches lesions, and forty-three cases of typhus fever. In the paper Jenner presented the results of his analysis to prove that the symptoms of the two fevers were generally different, that their characteristic eruptions, described as rose spots and a mulberry rash respectively, were diagnostic. All cases diagnosed as typhus on the basis of symptoms failed to show the lesions of Louis. Finally, Jenner established that while the epidemic constitution, as indicated by the relative frequency of the various forms, had changed repeatedly during the period of study, the results of the distinction, clinically and pathologically, remained constant.[41]

The fourth criterion, that in no circumstances was one disease ever transformed into the other, nor did the one ever produce a case of the other, Jenner made the subject of a special paper read to the Royal Medical and Chirurgical Society on 11 December 1849. In this paper Jenner followed the lead of William Henderson and described situations in which more than one case of febrile disease came from the same location. He used the diagnostic specificity established in his clinical pathological correlation to differentiate fever into three forms. In 1847 Jenner found twelve cases of typhus from five houses, four cases of typhoid fever from two houses, and ten cases of relapsing fever from five houses. "During the same time not a single example was observed of either disease communicating the other, or of cases of the three diseases, or even two of them, being generated by the same cause."[42]

Jenner further extended Henderson's method for the years 1848 and 1849, comparing the proportion of cases in his multi-case situation to the general proportions of the diseases in the London Fever Hospital population, further undermining the idea of an epidemic constitution. While he acknowledged the limited nature of his sample, Jenner was unable "to detect any hygienic differences in the condition of the people, or in the localities themselves to modify the exciting cause." The continued fevers were specific diseases, dependent on unique and specific causes for their production.

Jenner's conclusion was not immediately adopted by the entire British medical profession, but his demonstration of epidemiological specificity in combination with clinical and pathological differences convinced a significant proportion of British physicians. It had a definite influence in the United States and France, but most importantly it established the distinction in terms that were important to practitioners in Britain, so that Jenner was rightfully recognized as having achieved something not done by previous workers. His third publication, a series of twenty-one papers on the bedside appearances of the diseases previously called continued fevers, provided practitioners with a useful resource on clinical variations from the general clinical patterns. It was frequently compared to Pierre Louis's work on typhoid fever in terms of its precision and comprehensive nature.[43]

During the early 1850s, for reasons that are not at all clear, William Budd made no contribution to the debate over the identity or nonidentity of continued fevers. Perhaps Budd thought that Jenner's work was definitive and had preempted anything that he might have to offer on the subject. More likely, he did not have sufficient new information to warrant a publication on fever and was busily at work on the study of cholera, a subject on which he had data and which also illustrated the idea of specific contagion, for in 1847 Budd had an experience that altered his ideas on the mode of transmission of disease.

In 1847 Budd was called to see a patient with fever in Richmond Terrace, Clifton, a suburb of Bristol. He diagnosed the fever as typhoid and suspected there would be more than one case. He soon realized that there was a minor epidemic among the homes of Richmond Terrace, although among the thirty-four houses only thirteen experienced fever, at least one case occurring in each. The only connection among the thirteen houses was their common use of a well. In twenty-one other houses with different water supplies no fever occurred. In addition, there were at Clifton two girls' schools, one of which possessed an independent supply of water, whereas the other used the tainted pump. In the latter school, eleven of seventeen girls developed typhoid fever; in the former, there were no cases. Budd believed the well to have been poisoned by the specific cause of typhoid fever but could not establish how that might have happened. As a result, he did not publish his ideas but realized that it was possible to spread typhoid fever through water as well as through the air.[44]

In common with other public health reformers, Budd had urged effective sewers and pure water for the city of Bristol. In 1846 the Bristol Water Company was organized to provide pure water under constant pressure. William Budd was one of the directors. He believed that water quality was improving, so that, when in 1849 cholera struck Bristol, while he was prepared to accept the water-borne nature of some cases, he still believed strongly that the disease was spread principally through the air.

From his experiences with typhoid fever at North Tawton and Richmond Terrace, William Budd was able to analyze the epidemic pattern in cholera in the valley of the Avon River upstream from Bristol. He traced the spread into the small towns of Brightley Bridge and South Brent by people who had been infected with the disease at Plymouth and to his own satisfaction established that cholera was, like typhoid, a contagious disease spread through contaminated water. He published his theory of water transmission shortly after that of John Snow appeared, but Budd's ideas were independent.[45]

During the 1849 cholera epidemic Budd became involved in a controversy over the etiological agent of the disease. Several Bristol physicians, Budd among them, thought they had identified a fungus constantly associated with cholera and possibly the cause of the disease. Because his epidemiology had prepared him to accept a living disease-causing agent, he subscribed to the fungus theory and presented it with great vigor, but the cholera fungus proved short lived in medical science. Budd never again identified the exact nature of the causative agent of infectious diseases; he only described the properties that such causative agents must have epidemiologically.[46]

In the early 1850s Budd confined his attention to the practice of medicine in Bristol, publishing one clinical paper on brain abscess in 1851 and another on therapeutics in croup in 1852. He did teach his Bristol colleagues to distinguish typhoid from typhus fever. Typhoid was endemic in Bristol and typhus occurred only in epidemics among the Irish immigrants. When it occurred, the patients were almost always seen at St. Peter's Hospital, and Budd would invite colleagues from the Royal Infirmary to the hospital to see the second fever.[47]

In 1854 cholera again threatened Britain, and Budd published, at first anonymously, suggestions on how to prevent its spread by disinfection of intestinal discharges and the maintenance of pure water supplies.

The suggestions were sensible and proposed no definite etiological theory. The early papers were so well received that Budd admitted authorship in the latter part of the series, which he published under his own name.[48]

In the mid-1850s Budd received qualified support from William Alison and Thomas Watson, and by 1855 he may have felt somewhat more secure about reentering the debates on fever.[49]

By 1855 it had also become obvious that the battle was not over; powerful voices remained opposed to the work of William Jenner. Among the most influential may have been Thomas Addison, who could accept the distinction drawn among the various forms of continued fever only "provisionally in default of any more practical solution of the difficulty." On 15 November 1856 an account of fever at the clergy orphan school in St. John's Wood appeared in the *Lancet*. It excited interest because the school was generally healthy and "the most scrupulous attention to cleanliness" had been observed. When the students returned from the holidays, one was taken ill on 14 September. Within three weeks four other cases occurred, and at one point early in October, within one thirty-six-hour period seventeen students were taken ill. The reporter for the *Lancet* concluded, "The simultaneous seizure of the patients is sufficient to set aside the idea of contagion." Work done on the drains during the holiday was blamed for the outbreak.[50]

Such an account was like a red flag to William Budd, and, in a brief paper published on 6 December 1856, he explained the outbreak at St. John's Wood. First, he diagnosed the disease as *intestinal* or typhoid fever. He compared the events to those of other schools, the model for such outbreaks being that at the French military school at La Flèche in 1826. He explained briefly the role of diarrheal discharges in spreading the disease through either air or water and pointed out that the fever could be arrested by chemical disinfection of the discharges. Three weeks later an editorial by Budd on the contagiousness of typhoid fever appeared in the *Lancet;* he acknowledged the opposition of the Board of Health and the Royal College of Physicians to his strict contagionist views and gave a brief summary of his North Tawton experience, promising a more extensive account in the future.[51]

Yet Budd did not follow through, although he had been revising his account of the 1839 experience since 1842 at least. In 1858 the final spur was applied when Charles Murchison put forward the pythogenic theory of fever causation. Murchison received an M.D. at Edinburgh in 1851 and, after a postgraduate tour of hospitals and brief service with the East

India Company, settled in London. In 1855 he was appointed an assistant physician at the London Fever Hospital where, under the tutelage of William Jenner, he came to appreciate the distinctions among continued fevers that had been achieved by the numerical methods of Pierre Louis.[52]

Charles Murchison appreciated the "fact" that specific disease required specific causes; the vague multi-factoral hypotheses of earlier generations and the belief of the General Board of Health that smell was disease were both untenable. There was, however, an undeniable relationship between defective sewers and the spread of the typhoid fever. There were many cases of the disease in which direct sources of contagion could not be identified. Murchison constructed a composite, based on the organic chemistry of Justus Leibig, that resolved these anomalies. Pythogenic fever was the result of a particular poison produced by a specific form of putrefaction. The reason for the communicability of the fever was believed to be that the intestinal discharges of former fever patients were more likely to undergo the putrefaction that produced the specific poison than was normal sewage, but under the proper conditions, normal sewage could produce the poison and the disease could arise spontaneously. Murchison's theory was well received and represented a consensus opinion based on the sanitary reform experience and scientific researches on fever.[53]

In 1859 Budd published his extensive study of intestinal or typhoid fever, bringing together his epidemiological and pathological evidences and an understanding of scientific reasoning not shared by his contemporaries. He held that all situations in which the cause of a disease could not be identified provided only negative evidence, and no number of such cases could challenge good, positive evidence of contagion. Such a strict contagionist view was held by relatively few medical men. He also elaborated the definition of contagion to eliminate the need for direct contact; so long as there was a unique, material cause that had its origins in a former case, the disease was said to have spread by contagion.

The principal evidence in Budd's favor derived from his careful epidemiological studies, none of which were more telling than his account of the North Tawton epidemic of 1839. To support his theory further, he also used other, more recent examples. In 1855, Miss R. of St. Michael's Hill, Bristol, took five young ladies to France. She and four of the ladies went to Paris, while one returned home early. In Paris, a resident of the hotel where they stayed died of fever the day they left; on their return to England all of the young ladies had fever. One was nursed by a servant, who became ill and was sent to the Bristol Royal Infirmary, where Budd diagnosed the illness as typhoid fever and traced its history. In 1858–59, fever broke out in a school at Cardiff. One young man returned to his farm home outside Bristol, where he communicated the disease to two of his sisters, to a servant, and to a hired nurse.[54]

Budd based his belief that the most virulent poison originated from the lesions of the Peyer's patches in the intestines of previous victims on the unique pathology. From his own as well as others' work, he knew that the lesions of the Peyer's patches were the unique feature of typhoid fever. Therefore, he reasoned, only slightly more carefully than many had done, that the intestines were an important, if not primary, site of the disease. This opinion was supported also by the symptoms of diarrhea and abdominal discomfort often associated with the disease. From his extensive postmortem experience Budd thought that the lesions in the early stages of the disease (a state rarely seen) resembled the pustules of smallpox, suggesting an analogy between the two diseases.[55] If the analogy was correct, then a minute quantity of the matter from the lesions of the Peyer's patches would produce typhoid fever, just as a minute amount of matter from smallpox pustules could produce inoculated smallpox. Therefore, alvine discharges might easily contaminate the air or water if great care were not taken in nursing the sick to disinfect and dispose of waste. If the disease was spread through air or water, it would seem as if it had arisen from miasmata. Budd described two carefully documented cases of sewage contamination of water that had resulted in the spread of typhoid fever — at Abbotsham Place, Bristol, and at Richmond Terrace, Clifton.[56] He suggested that the material presented in the 1859–60 papers was essentially the same as that submitted for the Thackeray Prize in 1840, but there are substantial differences. By 1859 Budd differentiated fevers much more clearly and had developed his theory of the water-borne transmission. Nevertheless, there are striking parallels between the 1859 papers and the 1839 essay that reveal a definite continuity in his ideas over the twenty-year period.

The reaction to Budd's extensive articles of 1859–60 varied from a simple refusal to consider his ideas to a wholehearted acceptance, but most influential practitioners at least recognized his careful observations and gave them qualified acceptance. At one extreme W. Carmichael McIntosh, physician to the Perth Asylum, ignored facts supportive of Budd's theory. "The Epidemic [at the asylum] occurred in the Spring of 1862 and from all I can learn had no connection with the contagion, and indeed the onset of the fever in individual cases had little evidence of this

except in the instance of the man who waited on the male patients." The
first victim was a female attendant, followed by two patients whom she
worked with, and there were two or three other female patients who had
mild attacks that were diagnosed as ague. There were also several male
patients and one male attendant, who was considered the only case of
contagion, "for he not only occasionally waited on the male patients during the day, he slept in the same room at night." [57] Dr. McIntosh held a
concept of contagion obviously different from and considerably more
narrow than that of William Budd.

In his third report as medical officer of the Privy Council, John
Simon wrote:

> The facts which Dr. Budd adduces from his own experience and
> from that of other observers are, in my opinion, sufficient to prove
> that the contagium of typhoid fever is importable by persons who
> have the disease: . . . . And his arguments are also, I think, cogent
> to this general effect — that specially the bowel-discharges of the
> disease are means (yet not therefore necessarily the sole means) by
> which a patient, whether migrating or stationary, can be instrumen-
> tal in spreading the infection of typhoid fever. Provisionally these
> conclusions must be acted upon in their present unqualified form. [58]

Simon's understanding of the implications of Budd's findings was
reflected in his analysis of the epidemic of typhoid in Kingston-Deverill,
about which he concluded, "As regards the two chief media through
which intestinal contagions are too often filthily diffused — the medium
of sewage-tainted drinking water, and the medium of sewage-tainted
breathing air — Kingston-Deverill might seem to be rather exceptionally
well off: . . . . Probably an essential evil was, that no precautions were
taken in dealing with the evacuations of the sick. . . ." [59]

The precautions needed, in Simon's opinion, were described in a
"General Memorandum" on the prevention of epidemic diseases that he
had prepared for popular use. The general public health measures of
Simon's program were to enforce the existing laws, get the best medical
advice available, and pay particularly close attention to known problem
areas. In addition it recognized that in some cases it was necessary to use
chemical disinfectants, particularly "where cholera or typhoid fever is in
a house, the privy requires to be disinfected." The water supply should
be examined; "especially where the disease is cholera, diarrhea or
typhoid fever, it is essential that no foul water be drunk." Cleanliness
was always very important, but special precautions were necessary when

dealing with infective discharges of typhoid and cholera patients, whose "bedding, clothing, towels, and other articles" should be disinfected, as should the evacuations themselves before being thrown into privies, drains, or cesspools. A procedure for disinfection was circulated with the memorandum.[60]

Other medical authorities were not willing to give Budd as much acceptance, even though they could not deny his observations. Thomas B. Peacock, physician to St. Thomas's Hospital, said in an 1862 clinical lecture,

> Facts of this kind [referring to house-to-house passage of typhoid] are, it is true, open to objections; for the patients being all exposed to the operations of the same causes, the disease may originate independently in each case. Occasionally, however, we find infected persons removed to houses or districts previously free from the disease, propagate it in the situation to which they are removed, and thus afford conclusive proofs of contagion; but such cases are undoubtedly very rare, and generally the disease arises from defective sewage arrangements and exposure to decomposing animal matters.[61]

Country medical practitioners seem to have been more understanding of Budd's ideas than their city brothers. In response to Dr. Peacock's lecture, Dr. William Cook Low of Mortly, Worcester, wrote to the editor of the *Lancet* a letter in which he traced a country epidemic very similar to the North Tawton one of 1839 and argued that such cases were not at all rare. Similarly, Charles W. Whitby, M.B., of Ottery St. Mary, traced an 1862 epidemic from a girls' school into homes in his practice and from the children through the families. He did not know the original cause of the epidemic, but "whatever may have been the exciting cause of the first appearance of the fever it seems to me that the important fact that typhoid fever is, at times at least, highly infectious, is clearly proved in these cases."[62]

Most of these men could understand the advantage of Budd's ideas for practical medicine. Budd wrote, "For the emergence of actual fever, I have specific measures to propose, which come nearer to the root of the evil. By treating the intestinal discharges and everything imbued with them (including the hands of attendants on the sick), with proper disinfectant, I endeavor to stay the spread of the malady by destroying the very seed from which it sprung."[63]

Budd apparently was stating an argument that was convincing to at least some of his contemporaries, for in addition to Simon's memorandum, the Associated London Medical Officers of Health, in 1864, asked that the powers of the Disease Prevention Act include the provision that "local authorities should be required to provide appropriate means for the disinfection, by heat or otherwise, of bedding, clothes, etc." of patients suffering from infectious diseases, particularly typhoid fever and cholera.[64]

During the 1860s, Budd further elaborated his ideas in opposition to Murchison's pythogenic theory but could not compile enough evidence to convince his contemporaries that his was a complete explanation of the epidemiological phenomena associated with typhoid fever. As a result, he expanded his epidemiological researches to include epizootic diseases and drew parallels to human epidemics. He also wrote on other human infectious diseases — yellow fever, diphtheria, malignant pustule, phthisis, and scarlet fever.[65]

More importantly, during the 1860s Budd's ideas began to bear fruit, first in Bristol but also in other locations. In April 1864 typhus fever broke out at Bristol and by autumn had reached epidemic proportions. In 1865 John Simon sent Dr. George Buchanan to investigate the epidemic for the Privy Council, and Buchanan recommended the appointment of a medical officer of health to advise the local health board. By the 1848 Public Health Act, medical officers of health were permitted but not required, and most local authorities preferred not to employ one for reasons of economy. At Bristol Dr. David Davies was appointed medical officer of health in February 1865 and, by isolation of typhus fever patients and disinfection of their clothing, bedding, etc., brought the fever under control. Davies firmly believed in William Budd's suggestion for controlling epidemic disease, and in 1866, when cholera struck Bristol, there were only 49 cases. In September 1866 typhus fever again broke out in Bristol, but isolation and disinfection controlled the spread of the epidemic.[66]

In 1873 William Budd collected together his various papers and observations on fever in his classic monograph, *Typhoid Fever*. The book could do no more than the papers had done. There were many questions yet to answer. Great progress had been made since his initial effort in 1840; more research was still needed, but it would be done without William Budd. In 1873 he suffered a stroke and retired from practice. He died in 1880.

One problem Budd's theories of infection still had to overcome was that they were inadequate to explain all the typhoid fever of Britain. In

1870 T. Clifford Allbutt recognized a part of the problem when he wrote that most accounts of typhoid outbreaks did not trace the origin of the specific poison but were content to prove the fecal contamination of drinking water. Allbutt knew, as did almost everyone else, that drinking water contaminated with sewage was not good for people, but that in and of itself, such contamination did not produce typhoid fever — there were many known cases of tainted water without typhoid outbreaks. He further recognized that the problem of air contamination was unsolved and probably unsolvable. He doubted whether water would "cover all cases" and recognized that it was particularly difficult to explain in "large towns . . . where the water supply is uniform, continuous, and excellent, and where enteric fever is nevertheless prevalent." [67]

In a paper read before the South Midland branch of the British Medical Association in October 1868, Dr. Charles E. Prior of St. Peters, Bedford, noted part of the problem in saying:

> Many of these outbreaks (of enteric fever) may be accounted for on
> the explanation of Dr. Budd — namedly, the transmission by the
> sewers of the poison from intestinal discharge. Some of
> them, . . . have been a matter of question as to whether they were
> fever at all. There still however, remains a puzzling
> residuum. . . . Experience . . . gives a certain proportion of cases in
> which the disease could not be traced to contagion and appeared of
> spontaneous origin, children in the cradle being in two or three
> instances the first to be attacked and the disease spreading from
> them. [68]

As early as 1858 Michael Waistell Taylor of Penrith suggested that fevers might be communicated by ingested foods, but his paper seems to have attracted little attention. Part of the reason may have been that only once in a dozen pages did he name the fever with which he was concerned, and he then called it typhus. Thirty years later, in 1888, Richard Thorne believed that, in fact, Taylor was describing typhoid, and on the basis of the characteristics of the two diseases, Thorne's diagnosis was very probably correct. [69] It was left for Edward Ballard to relate typhoid fever to milk in 1870.

Edward Ballard had for fourteen years been medical officer to the parish of St. Mary, Islington, when typhoid broke out in epidemic proportions in 1870. After eliminating the common causes of the outbreak, he turned his attention gradually to milk. He had a long-standing interest in problems of the digestive system and the adulteration of foodstuffs. In a brilliant report, Ballard showed that of 140 families supplied by one dairy, there were 70 cases of typhoid (out of 168), 30 of which were fatal.[70] In 1872 his demonstration of the transmissibility of typhoid fever in milk was confirmed by M. K. Robinson in a typhoid fever epidemic at Leeds and by J. B. Russell at Glasgow in 1873.

Dr. Russell thought the case at Glasgow had established the desirability, under the Public Health Act, of requiring the removal of sick members of the family of a merchant to a hospital or of closing the shop to insure the purity of the merchandise, particularly foodstuffs.[71]

In April 1873 John Dougall, M.D., discussed milk infections before the sanitary section of the Philosophical Society of Glasgow. Since, he said, there were those who believed zymotic poisons were generated spontaneously in milk, he demonstrated that "zymotic contagia are not generated in milk *de novo* but . . . that unfermented milk is a favorable soil for their propagation." The question at issue then became how the milk became infected with the poison, and the answer was from either impure water or impure air. Dr. Dougall was not willing to decide, however, whether the impurity was necessarily a specific poison from a previous case of the disease.[72]

The theory of the spontaneous origin of fever had captured the minds of most medical practitioners so completely that Budd's arguments to the contrary were of little avail. Nevertheless, the value of his rules was continually recognized. In 1869 he contributed to the *British Medical Journal* a statement, "How to Prevent Typhoid Fever from Spreading," based on the assumption that alvine discharges infected the air, bed and body linens, and privies, cesspools, and drains. The rules consisted, like those of Simon, of good sanitary practice and the liberal use of disinfectants. These were described by the editor as having been "shown effectual in preventing spread of fatal typhoid," and he further suggested that they could be issued as a placard in areas where typhoid fever had become epidemic because of the neglect of proper sanitary measures.[73] The 1874 publication by the Manchester and Salford Sanitary Association entitled "Typhoid Fever: How To Avoid It, and To Prevent Its Spread" shows the effect Budd's theories exerted slowly on public health, but even in the mid-1870s they were not accepted fully.

An example of partial acceptance was the work of Surgeon Page of H.M. Sixth Dragoons at Newbridge Barracks, County Kildare, Ireland, in 1874. Page arrived at the barracks after an epidemic of typhoid had begun. He suspected that the source was the water supply, which was new and coincided with the outbreak. Analysis showed the water to be pure. Page recommended the isolation of fever patients in the contagion

Manchester and Salford Sanitary Association.

TYPHOID FEVER:
HOW TO AVOID IT, AND TO PREVENT ITS SPREAD.

THIS complaint, which is often called Gastric Fever, is a very serious disease. It is attributable, almost entirely to defective drainage, or to impure water. The poison by which it is diffused is chiefly contained in the discharges from the bowels of affected persons, and these discharges may infect—(1) the air, (2) the bed and body linen of the patient, (3) the privy and cesspool and the drains proceeding from them. From the latter source, the poison may soak through the soil into wells and affect the drinking water. If there is any wastepipe or other channel by which vapours can get from the sewers to cisterns or to other receptacles of drinking water, the poison may find its way along it and do great mischief.

A.—HOW TO AVOID IT.

1. *By proper drainage.* If any stench arises from the drains outside or inside the house, they are not perfect and require immediate attention. It would be well also for every one to make sure that the drains of his house are perfect.

2. *By drinking pure water.* When there is any question as to the purity of the water supply, it should be filtered and boiled before use, and well or pump water should never be used without these precautions, when there is any privy or drain or collection of stagnant water in the immediate neighbourhood.

3. *By disinfectants.* Fresh air is an excellent disinfectant, and should be allowed to circulate freely through the house by keeping open the doors, windows, and chimneys; and some of the undermentioned disinfectants should at intervals be put down the privies or closets and drains, and into the ash-pits.

B.—TO PREVENT ITS SPREAD.

1. The cause of the outbreak must be ascertained and removed.

2. The patient, if not removed to Hospital, must be placed in a large well-ventilated apartment, both for his own sake and on account of those around him.

3. To disinfect the air, place in the room and about the house basins containing Chloride of Lime and water, to which a few drops of Sulphuric Acid should be added at intervals.

4. The discharges from the bowels must be disinfected at once and before they are carried from the sick-room—for this purpose, Mc.Dougall's or Calvert's Powder, or one part of Carbolic Acid in 50 of water* should be put into the bed-pan every time before it is used by the patient, and a little of the Powder should be dredged into soiled spots on the linen.

5. All articles of bed or body-linen should be plunged immediately on removal, into a bucket containing a weak solution of Chloride of Lime, Disinfecting Powder, or Carbolic Acid. They should then be boiled before being washed.

6. As the hands of those attending the sick often become soiled with infectious matter, they should be frequently washed with one of the above solutions.

7. The privy or closet and all the drains should be flushed twice daily with the above-mentioned solution of Carbolic Acid, or with a solution of Green Vitriol (i.e., Sulphate of Iron) in the proportion of 1½lb. of the salt to a gallon of water.

8. In towns and villages where the fever is prevalent, this last rule should be put in force in all houses, whether there be fever in them or not, and all public drains should be flushed with disinfectants.

9. At the termination of the case, whether by death or recovery, the bedding, as well as the linen and clothing of both patient and nurses, should be taken to the Disinfecting Ovens, and the room should be fumigated by Chlorine or the fumes of burning Sulphur.

10. In the event of death, the corpse should be placed in a coffin as soon as possible, and sprinkled with Disinfecting Powder. Early burial is also most desirable.

* Suitable Disinfectants may be had at the Town Halls of Manchester and Salford ; and clothing, bedding, houses, &c., will be disinfected safely, and without charge, upon application at the respective Health Offices.

Issued by the Committee of the Manchester and Salford Sanitary Association, 78, Cross Street, Manchester.
September, 1874.   *May also be had on Cardboard, price one halfpenny each.*

POWLSON AND SONS, PRINTERS, SOUTH KING STREET, MANCHESTER.

wards of Hare Park Hospital and insisted on the disinfection, with chloride of zinc, of the "dejecta and discharges from the patients." He then traced the source of the epidemic to an unventilated sewage disposal system, which caused a concentration of effluvia to be built up and to be forced back into the houses. He could find no impure food or water, and since the cases were not localized, he could not support "direct contaga" (i.e., from person to person). He believed sewer emanations were capable of exciting the disease and when the sewer was ventilated the epidemic was finally brought under control.[74]

A decision between the theories of Budd and Murchison was not considered to be necessary or even desirable by some members of the medical profession. When, in 1874, Dr. William Strange of Worcester wrote in the *Medical Times and Gazette* to urge medical officers of health, particularly, to subscribe to the pythogenic theory of the origin of typhoid, he was answered by an editorial that denied the validity or necessity of choosing. For the editor, "the practical application of either theory does not in the slightest degree interfere with the working of the other, rather they serve to complement one another." They complemented each other in that the pythogenic theory necessitated the careful control of water supply and drainage while Budd's required every precaution to stop the spread of the disease, particularly by disinfection.[75]

A summary of opinion concerning typhoid in 1874 may be found in Simon's supplementary report, "Filth-Diseases and their Prevention." He states his theory of typhoid as:

> Since the year 1849, when Dr. (now Sir William) Jenner made known his conclusive and masterly discrimination of this specific form of fever, successive studies have tended with singular uniformity to connect it in regard to its origin with nuisances of an excremental sort [the work of Murchison] . . . the explanation of the frequent but not invariable tendency of privy-nuisances to infect with enteric fever, has seemed to consist in the ability of such nuisances to carry with them, not invariably, but as frequent accidental adjunct, the "specific" contagium of any prevailing bowel infection [the work of Budd]. . . . Medical knowledge in support of this presumption has of late been rapidly growing more positive and precise; [Simon believed that Dr. Klein had isolated a specific enteric fever microphyte].

Then Simon gave his administrative position: "In order to reduce that vast quantity of preventable disease which has its type in enteric fever, and in relation to which each individual case of enteric fever which occurs ought to be regarded as having an important local significance, the one essential condition is CLEANLINESS." As for disinfection, "to chemically disinfect the filth of every neglected district . . . cannot . . . be proposed as physically possible. . . . This opinion . . . does not at all discredit the appeals which are constantly and very properly made to chemistry . . . with regard, . . . to the management of individual cases of infectious disease and to the immediate disinfection of everything which comes from them."[76]

Very few medical practitioners thought that Budd's theory of the contagion of typhoid fever was correct. Contingent contagionist theories were deeply entrenched in Britain and were believed to have been confirmed by the success of public health reform. The original surveys of the health of the British were made by men like Thomas Southwood Smith who "knew" fever to be the result of the body's natural defenses being overcome by exposure to an ill-defined, but powerful, poison. With the creation of Edwin Chadwick's General Board of Health, the equation of filth with disease was carried to extremes that the medical profession itself was not prepared to support. Some balance was regained with the appointment of John Simon as medical officer to the Privy Council of Britain and with the more scientifically formulated opinions of physicians such as Charles Murchison.

Despite John Snow's and his own work on cholera, William Budd did not have a sufficient body of evidence to support his theory of contagion. There were very definitely cases of infection that his theory could not explain. The immune carrier concept was still two generations away. Furthermore, the framework of scientific medicine could not easily accommodate theories of contagion before the germ theory was established. The typhoid bacillus was not isolated until 1880, the year of Budd's death.

While Budd considered the spontaneous generation of life a closed question, it was, in reality, still unsettled in the early 1870s. As long as serious scientists continued to believe in the possibility of the spontaneous origin of life, the arguments for the spontaneous origin of disease were not nearly so unsupportable as Budd liked to claim. The chemistry of fermentation, only then being developed, suggested the real possibility of the creation of specific substances in decomposing animal matter — substances that might serve as a specific typhoid poison. It was only in the late 1870s that John Tyndall settled the spontaneous generation problem with his "optically empty" chamber experiments. The work of

Tyndall and Ferdinand Cohn on *Bacillus subtilus* prepared the way for a new germ theory based in bacteriology.

In the light of such difficulties, that portion of Budd's work that was of obvious value to his contemporaries was his concept that the intestinal discharges were the most dangerous sources of future infections and his insistence on the need to disinfect them chemically. The concept and practice depended upon the recognition of typhoid fever as a unique disease with a specific cause. For William Budd, this recognition came at North Tawton in 1839, but for the majority of the medical profession, the careful *urban* epidemiological distinctions of William Jenner were the deciding factor. In the 1850s, after the work of Jenner, Budd's ideas were recognized as valuable quite soon after he published them, and his recommendations rapidly became a standard epidemic control measure. Yet to use Budd's research in sanitary measures did not require the full acceptance of his ideas, an act of faith that most Victorian medical practitioners would have considered unscientific, if not irrational. Only in such a limited application as the practice of disinfection could Budd's work have been of immediate assistance in the control of typhoid fever, and in this way, after 1860, it probably was. This limited value was not to be found in the Thackeray Prize essay of 1840, so that, while it was and is interesting, it was not sufficiently developed in 1840 to exercise an impact on Victorian medicine.

NOTES

1. Budd manuscript, p. 179; my emphasis.

2. William Budd to Richard Budd, 11 January 1841 and 7 November 1842, Budd Letters, Wellcome Institute, London.

3. A. P[richard], "William Budd, F.R.S.," *Bristol R. Infir. Rep.*, 1878-79, *1*, 361.

4. Budd manuscript, p. 22.

5. Andrew Anderson, *Observations on Typhus* (Glasgow: J. Hedderwick and Son, 1840).

6. Alexander P. Stewart, "Some Considerations on the Nature and Pathology of Typhus and Typhoid Fever, Applied to the Solution of the Question of the Identity or Non-identity of the Two Diseases," *Edin. Med. Surg. J.*, 1840, *54*, 289-339.

7. "Continued Fevers of France and England," *Brit. For. Med. R.*, 1841, *12*, 293-326.

8. H. C. Barlow, "On the Distinction between Typhus Fever and Dothienenterie," *Lancet*, 1839-40, *1*, 838-41.

9. "Louis' Researches on Typhoid Fever," *Brit. For. Med. R.*, 1841, *12*, 22-53.

10. Dale C. Smith, "Medical Science, Medical Practice, and the Emerging Concept of Typhus in Mid Eighteenth Century Britain," in W. F. Bynum and V. Nutton, eds., *Theories of Fever From Antiquity to the Enlightenment* (London: Wellcome Institute, 1981), pp. 121-34.

11. Robert Christison, "Continued Fever," in Alexander Tweedie, ed., *A System of Practical Medicine*, 3 vols. (Philadelphia: Lea and Blanchard, 1842), 1, 136–98; Alexander Tweedie, "Fever" and "Fever, Continued," in John Forbes, et al., eds., *The Cyclopedia of Practical Medicine*, 4 vols. (Philadelphia: Lea and Blanchard, 1849), 2, 147–201.

12. Thomas Hodgkin, *Lectures on the Morbid Anatomy of the Serous and Mucous Membranes*, 2 vols. (London: Sherwood Gilbert and Piper, 1839–40), 2, 464.

13. "Continued Fevers," pp. 325–26.

14. William Farr, "Statistical Nosology," an appendix to the *Fourth Annual Report of the Registrar-General* (London: Her Majesty's Stationery Office, 1842), pp. 147–216. On Farr's development and use of this nosology see John M. Eyler, *Victorian Social Medicine: The Ideas and Methods of William Farr* (Baltimore: The Johns Hopkins University Press, 1979), pp. 52–60; and Margaret Pelling, *Cholera, Fever, and English Medicine 1825–1865* (Oxford: Oxford University Press, 1978), pp. 92–100. Farr did not change the official nosology until 1869, but did recognize the change in ideas of the mid-1850s. See Farr, "Report on Nomenclature and Classification" in the *Sixteenth Annual Report of the Registrar-General* (London: Her Majesty's Stationery Office, 1856), pp. 15–16.

15. Charles Murchison, *A Treatise on the Continued Fevers of Great Britain* (London: Parker and Bourn, 1862), pp. 47–48.

16. William P. Alison, "Remarks on the Present Epidemic," *Scot. Nth. Engl. Med. Gaz.*, 1843, *1*, 1–4.

17. William T. Gairdner, *The Physician as Naturalist: Addresses and Memoirs Bearing on the History and Progress of Medicine Chiefly during the Last Hundred Years* (Glasgow: Maclehose, 1889), pp. 396, 407–17, 424.

18. Benjamin Welsh, *Practical Treatise on the Efficacy of Bloodletting in the Epidemic Fever of Edinburgh* (Edinburgh: Bell and Bradfute, 1819); R. Christison, "On the Changes Which Have Taken Place in the Constitution of Fevers and Inflammations in Edinburgh, during the Last 40 years," *Edin. Med. J.*, 1858, *3*, 577–95.

19. W. R. Murray, "Destitution and Fever," *Scot. Nth. Eng. Med. Gaz.*, 1843, *1*, 164–67; William Reid, "The New Form of Fever at Present Prevalent in Scotland," *Lond. Med. Gaz.*, 1843, *33*, 358–62; Matthew H. Gibson, "Account of the Epidemic Fever Prevailing in Glasgow and Its Neighbourhood," *Lancet*, 1843–44, *1*, 330–34; William P. Alison, *Observations in the Epidemic Fever of 1843 in Scotland and Its Connection with the Destitute Conditions of the Poor* (Edinburgh, 1844); William Robertson, "Note on the Prevailing Fever," *Edin. Monthly J. Med. Sci.*, 1844, *4*, 110–12; Robert Jackson, "Account of the Epidemic Fever at Perth in 1843," *Edin. Med. Surg. J.*, 1844, *61*, 417–31; John Rose Cormack, *Natural History, Pathology, and Treatment of the Epidemic Fever at Present Prevailing in Edinburgh and Other Towns* (Edinburgh, 1843); J. Arrott, "Letter on the Present Epidemic of Dundee," *Scot. Nth. Eng. Med. Gaz.*, 1843, *1*, 129; William Henderson, "Clinical Observations on Fever," *Scot Nth. Eng. Med. Gaz.*, 1844, *1*, 162–64; Alexander Kilgour, "Remarks on the Epidemic Fever in Aberdeen during the Year 1843," *Scot. Nth. Eng. Med. Gaz.*, 1844, *1*, 321–23; David Smith, "Some Account of the Epidemic Fever Prevailing in Glasgow," *Edin. Med. Surg. Jr.*, 1844, *61*, 67–74; William Mackenzie, "Some Account of the Epidemic Remittent Fever Prevalent in Glasgow in 1843," *Lond. Med. Gaz.*, 1843, *33*, 225–36; A. Halliday Douglas, "Statistical Report of the Edinburgh Epidemic Fever of 1843–4," *Nthn. J. Med.*, 1844–45, *2*, 8, 209, 269; John Richard Wardell, *On the Scotch Epidemic Fever of 1843–4*, etc. (London, 1848).

20. David Craigie, "Notice of a Febrile Disorder Which Has Prevailed at Edinburgh During the Summer of 1843," *Edin. Med. Surg. J.*, 1843, *60*, 410–18.

21. Ibid., p. 417.

22. William Henderson, "On Some of the Characters Which Distinguish the Fever at Present Epidemic from Typhus Fever," *Edin. Med. Surg. J.*, 1844, *61*, 201-25.

23. Ibid., p. 202.

24. Ibid., p. 203.

25. Ibid., pp. 206-19.

26. Ibid., pp. 214-17.

27. Ibid., pp. 217-18.

28. Ibid., p. 219.

29. "Obituary. Sir William Jenner, Bart., M.D., F.R.C.P. Lond., F.R.S., etc." *Lancet*, 1898, *2*, 1674-76.

30. Thomas Watson, *Lectures on the Principles and Practice of Physic*, 3 vols., (London: Parker, 1843-44), *2*, 692.

31. William Budd, "On Intestinal Fever," *Lancet*, 1859, *2*, 4-5, 28-30, 55-56, 80-82, 131-33, 207-10, 432-33, 458-59; 1860, *1*, 187-90, 239-40.

32. Elisha Bartlett, *The History, Diagnosis and Treatment of Typhoid and of Typhus Fever* (Philadelphia: Lea and Blanchard, 1842); "Dr. Bartlett on Typhoid and Typhus Fever," *Brit. For. Med. Rev.*, 1844, *17*, 357-70.

33. Pelling, *Cholera, Fever, and English Medicine*, pp. 1-80.

34. William Jenner, *Lectures and Essays on Fevers and Diphtheria 1849 to 1879* (London: Rivington, Percival, 1893), p. 167; the physician was quite probably Robert Carswell of University College, with whom Jenner continued to do pathological work after graduation in 1844.

35. Alexander Duncan, *Memorials of the Faculty of Physicians and Surgeons of Glasgow 1599-1850* (Glasgow: Maclehose, 1896), p. 282.

36. "Medical News. Medico-Chirurgical Society of Glasgow," *Monthly J. Med. Sci.*, 1846, *7*, 316-17.

37. Charles Ritchie, "Practical Remarks on the Continued Fevers of Great Britain and on the Generic Distinction between Enteric Fever and Typhus," *Monthly J. Med. Sci.*, 1846, *7*, 247-58.

38. Ritchie's paper is cited by Leslie T. Morton, ed., *Garrison-Morton, A Medical Bibliography*, 4th ed. (London: Gower, 1983), item 5026, for introducing the term *enteric fever*, but the earliest citation I have found by contemporaries is in Charles Murchison's *Treatise on the Continued Fevers of Great Britain* (London, 1862), which contained a relatively complete but uncritical bibliography.

39. Edward Latham Ormerod, *Clinical Observations on the Pathology and Treatment of Continued Fever* (London: Longman, Brown, Green, and Longmans, 1848).

40. Jenner, *Fever*, pp. 4-6.

41. Ibid., p. 133.

42. Ibid., p. 149.

43. Dale C. Smith, "Gerhard's Distinction between Typhoid and Typhus and Its Reception in America, 1833-1860," *Bull. Hist. Med.*, 1980, *54*, 368-85; C. P. Forget, "Preuves cliniques de la non-identité du typhus et de la fièvre typhoïde," *Gaz. Méd. de Paris*, 1854, 3d. ser., *9*, 644, 659, 700, 714; Alexander P. Stewart in particular contested Jenner's claim to the distinction, but J. Warburton Begbie in his review, "Jenner and Flint on Typhus and Typhoid Fevers," *Brit. For. Med. Chir. Rev.*, 1855, *16*, 409-20, was probably correct in his appraisal: "The actual demonstration . . . remained for Dr. Jenner to accomplish."

44. Budd, "On Intestinal Fever," pp. 131–33, 207, 432.

45. William Budd, *Malignant Cholera: Its Cause, Mode of Propagation, and Prevention* (London: Churchill, 1849).

46. Ibid. and Pelling, *Cholera, Fever, and English Medicine*, pp. 146–202.

47. Budd, "On Intestinal Fever," p. 131.

48. William Budd [Common Sense, pseud.], "Cholera: Its Cause and Prevention," *Ass. Med. J.*, 1854, *2*, 928–29, 950–51; William Budd, "Cholera: Its Cause and Prevention," *Ass. Med. J.*, 1854, *2*, 974–78; 1855, *3*, 207–8, 283.

49. Pelling, *Cholera, Fever, and English Medicine*, pp. 46, 271.

50. "Dr. Addison on Dr. Jenner's views, [etc.]" *Ass. Med. J.*, 1856, *4*, 993; "Outbreak of Fever at the Clergy Orphan School in St. John's Wood," *Lancet*, 1856, *2*, 555.

51. William Budd, "On the Fever at the Clergy Orphan Asylum," *Lancet*, 1856, *2*, 617–19.; William Budd, "On Intestinal Fever: Its Mode of Propagation," *Lancet*, 1856, *2*, 694–95.

52. *Dictionary of National Biography*, s.v., "Murchison, Charles."

53. Charles Murchison, "Contributions to the Etiology of Continued Fever: Or an Investigation of Various Causes Which Influence the Prevalence and Mortality of Its Different Forms," *Med. Clin. Trans.*, 1858, *41*, 219–306; Pelling, *Cholera, Fever, and English Medicine*, pp. 287–92.

54. Budd, "On Intestinal Fever," p. 60.

55. On the use of exanthemata as an analogy in pathology and epidemiology see Pelling, *Cholera, Fever, and English Medicine* and Lloyd Stevenson, "A Pox on the Ileum," *Bull. Hist. Med.*, 1977, *51*, 496–504.

56. Budd, "On Intestinal Fever," p. 60.

57. W. Carmichael McIntosh, "Asylum Notes on Typhoid Fever," *J. Mental Sci.*, 1863–64, *9*, 24–36.

58. John Simon, *Third Report of the Medical Officer of the Privy Council, 1860* (London: Her Majesty's Stationery Office, 1861), p. 2, in the footnote.

59. Ibid., pp. 10–11.

60. Ibid., pp. 37–40.

61. Thomas B. Peacock, "On the Recent Epidemic of Fever," *Lancet*, 1862, *2*, 4–6.

62. William Cook Low, "Typhoid Fever Propagated by Contagion," *Lancet*, 1862, *2*, 93; Charles W. Whitby, "Is Typhoid Fever Infectious?" *Med. Times Gaz.*, 1862, *1*, 20–21.

63. William Budd, "Propagation of Typhoid Fever," *Lancet*, 1861, *2*, 533–34.

64. John Simon, *Seventh Report of the Medical Officer of the Privy Council, 1864* (London: Her Majesty's Stationery Office, 1865), p. 230.

65. William Budd, "On the Contagion of Yellow Fever," *Lancet*, 1861, *1*, 337–38; "Diphtheria," *Br. Med. J.*, 1861, *1*, 575–79; "On the Occurrence of Malignant Pustule in England," *Lancet*, 1862, *2*, 164–65; "Memorandum on the Nature and Mode of Propagation of Phthisis," *Lancet*, 1867, *2*, 451–52; "Scarlet Fever and Its Prevention," *Br. Med. J.*, 1869, *2*, 23–24. On his use of animal models see "Variola Ovina, Sheep's Smallpox; or the Laws of Contagious Epidemics Illustrated by an Experimental Type," *Br. Med. J.*, 1863, *2*, 142–50; "Investigation of Epidemic and Epizootic Diseases," *Br. Med. J.*, 1864, *2*, 354–57; "Observations on Typhoid (Intestinal) Fever in the Pig," *Br. Med. J.*, 1865, *2*, 81–87; "The Siberian Cattle-Plague; or, the Typhoid Fever of the Ox," *Br. Med. J.*, 1865, *2*, 169–79.

66. David Large and Frances Round, *Public Health in Mid-Victorian Bristol* (Bristol: The University, 1974), pp. 14–17.

67. Thomas C. Allbutt, "On the Propagation of Enteric Fever," *Brit. Med. J.*, 1870, *1*, 308-9.

68. Charles E. Prior, "On the Local and Spontaneous Origin of Enteric Fever," *Lancet*, 1870, *2*, 289-90, 327-29.

69. Michael Waistell Taylor, "On the Communication of the Infection of Fevers by Ingesta," *Edin. Med. Jr.*, 1858, *3*, 993-1004; Richard Thorne Thorne, *On the Progress of Preventive Medicine during the Victorian Era* (London: Shaw, 1888), p. 47.

70. Edward Ballard, *The Physical Diagnosis of Diseases of the Abdomen* (London: Taylor, Walton, & Maberly, 1852); idem, *On Pain after Food: Its Cause and Treatment* (London: Walton and Maberly, 1854); idem, *On Artificial Digestion* (London: Walton and Maberly, 1857); idem, *On an Outbreak of Typhoid Fever at Islington* (London: Churchill, 1871).

71. J. B. Russell, "Report on an Outbreak of Enteric Fever Connected with Milk Supply," *Glasgow Med. J.*, 1873, *5*, 474-81.

72. John Dougall, "On the Dissemination of Zymotic Diseases by Milk," *Glasgow Med. J.*, 1873, *5*, 312-31.

73. William Budd, "How to Prevent Typhoid Fever from Spreading," *Br. Med. J.*, 1869, *1*, 290.

74. [William John] Page, "Account of an Outbreak of Enteric Fever Which Occurred at Newbridge Barracks, County Kildare, 1874," in *Army Medical Department Reports, 1873* (London, 1875), pp. 301-3.

75. "The Nature and Origin of Typhoid Considered More Especially with Regard to Its Prevention and Treatment," *Med. Times Gaz.*, 1874, *2*, 215.

76. John Simon, *Report of the Medical Officer of the Privy Council and Local Government Board*, n.s., 2 (London: Her Majesty's Stationery Office, 1874), pp. 13-14, 26, 25.

APPENDIX:

THE NATIONAL LIBRARY OF MEDICINE ESSAY OF 1839 AND WILLIAM BUDD'S LATER WORK

There are several general similarities between the National Library of Medicine manuscript (MS/B/72) and Budd's later work. The title is very similar to the one that William Budd referred to later and differs only slightly from the essay question and Davidson's essay title. The manuscript begins with the title "An Essay On the Causes and Mode of Propagation of the Common Continued Fevers of Great Britain and Ireland," which corresponds closely to the title William Budd gave for his essay in 1859 — "essay on the 'Causes and Mode of Propagation of the Common Continued Fevers of Great Britain and Ireland.'"[1] The quotation used as an epigraph in the 1839 manuscript was from "Howard on Lazurettoes" — "If it were asked what is the cause of Jail fever? . . . I am obliged to look out for some additional cause of its production." In 1859 William Budd used the same quotation to head the third section of his paper, "Intestinal Fever."[2] In the 1839 essay the author refers repeatedly to his study with Pierre Louis; Budd was a Louis student. The author also refers to his experience at the "Seamen's Hospital" in the winter of 1838–39 (p. 111), the same time when William Budd was working there with his brother George.

The most important feature that establishes the NLM manuscript as William Budd's Thackeray Prize essay is the description of the fever epidemic in the village of North Tawton in 1839. The similarities seem to identify the manuscript as his beyond question. In Budd's 1859 description of this epidemic, the first case was of "Ann N_____, a young woman who was taken ill in the second week of July," while in the village epidemic of the NLM manuscript, the first case described was of "Ann Northam aged 16," who "began to droop the 8th July" and who was "laid up with fever on the 11th." The Northam household included the parents and four children, one of them a child two years old. Ann Northam's father, who had had the fever before, and the two-year-old were the only ones to escape it. Mrs. Northam and Ann's two sisters had it. In 1859 Budd described the North Tawton experience in which "the mother, a brother and a sister," of Ann N_____ caught the fever; "the father, who had already had the disease in former years, and a young infant," were the only family members spared.

There is a similar close, but not identical, account of the experience of two sawyers in the North Tawton epidemic. In the NLM manuscript the fourth case was a sawyer, Cheriton; the sixth, his mate, a sawyer named Allen. The 1839 account refers (p. 50) to the "fourth case, a sawyer" as having

> removed to his own home, nine miles off, soon after he began to droop. Two days after his return home he was laid up with fever of which he died at the end of 5 weeks. Ten days after his death his two children were also laid up with fever and both had it severely. The widow continued well.

In 1859 Budd describes the experience of the sawyers, who returned to their homes in the parish of Morchard "about seven miles off."

> The first, A_____ by name, was a married man, with two children. He left North Tawton on the 9th of August, being already too ill to work. Two days after reaching Morchard he took to his bed, and at the end of five weeks he died. Ten days after his death his two children were laid up with the same fever, and had it severely; the widow escaped.[3]

In the 1839 manuscript the sixth case was a sawyer, Allen, who on the ninth of August "felt unwell and removed to his own home." The further experience of Allen in the manuscript corresponds closely to that of the sawyer C_____ in William Budd's 1859 report. In both cases a friend came to visit the sick sawyer and, while assisting in raising the patient in the bed, was overcome by the putrid odor characteristic of typhoid patients; in both cases the friend continued to be bothered by a persistence of the odor for ten days following the incident, after which he was taken ill. The friend's two children, and a brother who frequently visited the house were in both reports also taken ill, while the elderly couple who lived with the sawyer in both reports escaped the disease.[4] The accounts are strikingly similar although one or the other account has the two sawyers confused. In 1859 William Budd acknowledged his indebtedness to Mr. Brutton, surgeon of Morchard, for the details reported; in the 1839 essay there is no such acknowledgment of outside assistance.

There is a further difference between Budd's later account and the manuscript that is of some significance because it plays an important role in the development of Budd's ideas. In the 1859 paper he wrote, "It was not until the summer before last that I first became aware that M. Bretonneau had put forward the same view in a paper, which was read to the French Academy of Medicine so long ago as July 7th, 1829."[5] Pierre Bretonneau reported on the 1826 epidemic of fever at the military school La Flèche at Tours, and his paper was printed in 1829. Budd's paper appeared in the summer of 1859 but he refers to the epidemic at the "military school of La Flèche, in France, in 1826," in his first communication on fever to the *Lancet*, December 1856;[6] so the date must be the summer of 1856, not 1857, and we must suppose that Budd was composing the long article on typhoid fever over a period of time prior to its submission to the *Lancet*. In the 1839 NLM manuscript the author is aware of and quotes the account of the military school epidemic from Bretonneau's 1829 paper (pp. 55-56). Nevertheless, the epidemic reported in the manuscript is clearly the one at North Tawton in 1839, which proves beyond reasonable doubt that the 1839 manuscript is William Budd's Thackeray Prize essay since he was the medical practitioner at North Tawton in 1839. Budd simply owed a greater debt to Pierre Bretonneau than he remembered in later years.

In 1859 Budd recalled that his Thackeray Prize essay "had three principal objects — The first was to prove, by various evidence, that the typhoid fever and the maculated typhus — the fever with intestinal affection, and the fever without such affection — are not varieties merely of one disease, but two diseases of essentially distinct species."[7] In the first chapter of the manuscript, the author set forth the problem that there were two "forms of essential fever, commonly called typhoid or typhous fever," which differed one from the other in that one had "that special alteration of the intestinal follicles, which on account of its constancy in Fever in Paris is there regarded as the anatomical character of the disease." Before discussing the question proposed by the Provincial Medical and Surgical Association — the causes and mode of propagation — the author of the 1839 essay thought it essential to establish that there existed two distinct fevers, the etiology and epidemiology of which would have to be considered separately.

The first evidence of specificity advanced was that the form of fever without alterations of the small bowel was never seen at Paris, or apparently at Boston. Just how the author knew of the study of typhoid fever led by James Jackson at the Massachusetts General Hospital is unclear.

There are several possibilities. In the preface to his 1836 English translation of Louis's monograph on typhoid fever, Henry Ingersol Bowditch suggested that the fever experiences of Boston and Paris were comparable. In American medical periodicals as well as in James Jackson's *Memoir* of his son there were various published accounts of the study of typhoid fever at Boston. Budd might have learned of the Boston work indirectly in the 1839 accounts of Louis's French student François Valleix. More probably he learned of it directly either at Paris from Pierre Louis or, even more likely, from George Cheyne Shattuck, who was in London in February and March 1839 and may have met Budd at either the London Fever Hospital or the *Dreadnought,* the seamen's hospital. Such hearsay communication is suggested further by the author's knowledge, indicated in his original n. (33), of the existence of James Jackson's *Report on Typhoid Fever* (1838) although he had never seen a copy.

The author realized that, while the absence of fever without intestinal affection in some locations strongly suggested that it was a specific disease, there were other possible explanations. He thought that "differences of climate, . . . diet, and . . . other conditions still more vague and indefinite" were inadequate because there had been French epidemics of fever without lesions and the English did have some cases of fever with lesions. His easy dismissal of such explanations reflected his previous commitment to the specific nature of typhoid fever, for careful practitioners knew that experimental proof was necessary. When James Jackson, Jr. first wrote to his father about the constant finding of intestinal lesions in Paris, the senior Jackson, like many British practitioners, suggested that therapeutic differences, particularly the French neglect of purgatives in fever, might explain the difference. The younger Jackson took his father's suggestion to Gabriel Andral, who responded, "Perhaps, sir, but a series of experiments with purgatives in Paris is necessary to prove it."[8]

Following the pattern and methods of Louis, the author of the manuscript then turned his attention to secondary characteristics of the two diseases that he believed further supported their specificity. First was the greater tendency to form "ulcerations on membranous tissue generally" observed in the Paris form of fever. Second was the difference in the cutaneous eruption. In the fever without intestinal lesions the spots were "not only more frequent, but also much more numerous"; it was frequently described as "measles like" and generally appeared earlier in the course of the disease than did the rose-colored spots described by Louis.

In fairness the author then drew attention to the similarities between the two forms of fever but argued that such similarities were shared, to one degree or another, by many acute diseases. They were, therefore, of little value in resolving the question of specificity and were greatly outweighed in the pathological study of the diseases by the differences between the two forms. Yet the issue was not absolutely settled by postmortem or symptomatic differences, no matter how great. The essential evidence was epidemiological. "If these forms be mere varieties of one disease it necessarily follows that one communicates the other. . . . It is for those who have opportunities of observation in places where both forms are common to determine, whether or not this be the case" (p. 22). The author thought that the answer was predictable as a result of experience at Paris, where the form of fever with intestinal lesions was common but where the other was unknown. He concluded the first chapter, "We are at present bound to act . . . in all that related to these forms of fever, to consider them as different diseases."

The second and third objectives of Budd's Thackeray Prize essay were to establish "that both species are essentially contagious [and] that there is no valid evidence to show that the specific poison from which either respectively springs is ever bred elsewhere than in the living and already infected body, but every reason to believe, on the contrary, that both are propagated by the law of continuous succession."[9] The second and third chapters of the NLM manuscript undertook to demonstrate the contagious character of each form of fever, in chapter two of the fever with intestinal lesions and in chapter three of the form without such lesions. The bulk of the essay is the second chapter (pp. 25–149) because the fever dealt with was "the only form of typhoid fever which occurrs in that part of England in which I reside; in rural districts at least."

These similarities to Budd's later publications, as well as the close correspondence between the NLM essay and Budd's own abstract of his Thackeray Prize essay in his letter to George Budd of 6 December 1839,[10] are sufficient to establish beyond any reasonable doubt that the NLM manuscript is William Budd's "lost" Thackeray Prize essay.

NOTES

1. William Budd, "On Intestinal Fever," *Lancet*, 1859, *2*, 4–5, 28–30, 55–56, 80–82, 131–33, 207–10, 432–33, 458–59; 1860, *1*, 187–90, 239–40.

2. Ibid., p. 432.

3. Ibid., p. 28.

4. Ibid., pp. 28–29 and the manuscript, pp. 51–52.

5. Budd, "On Intestinal Fever," p. 209.

6. William Budd, "On the Fever at the Clergy Orphan Asylum," *Lancet,* 1856, *2,* 617–19.

7. Budd, "On Intestinal Fever," p. 5.

8. James Jackson, *A memoir of James Jackson, Jr., M.D.* (Boston: I. R. Butts, 1835), pp. 120–21.

9. Budd, "On Intestinal Fever," p. 5.

10. Quoted in the text, p. 31 above.

INDEX

161

Lightning Source UK Ltd.
Milton Keynes UK
UKOW02f1435260914

239218UK00002B/164/A